COMPLETE Essential Oil DIFFUSER RECIPES

Over 150 Recipes for Health and Wellness

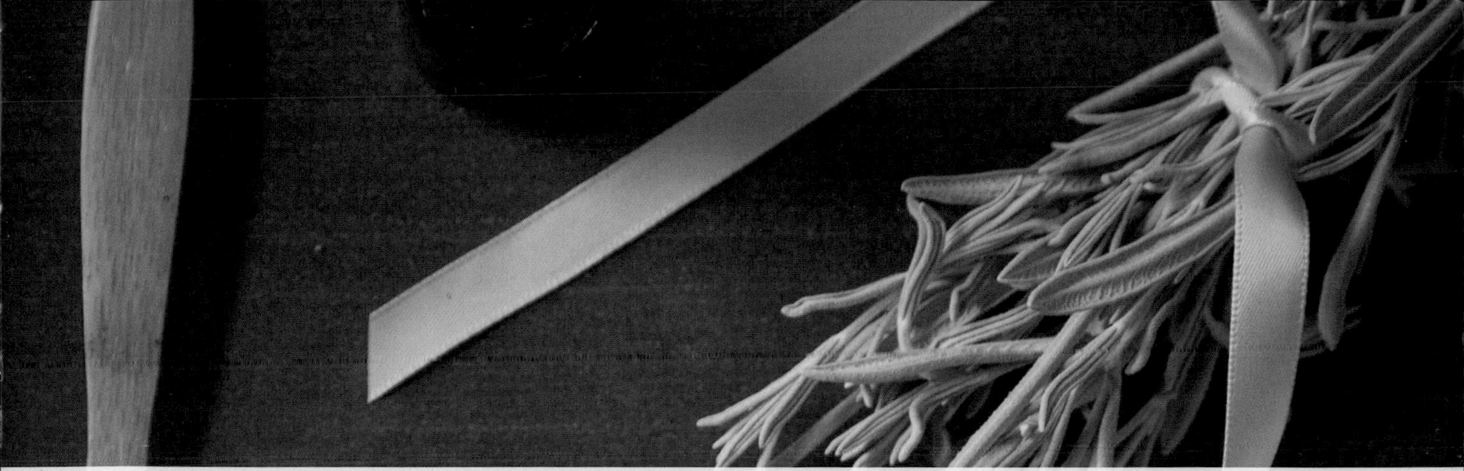

COMPLETE

Essential Oil

DIFFUSER RECIPES

Over 150 Recipes for Health and Wellness

PAM FARLEY

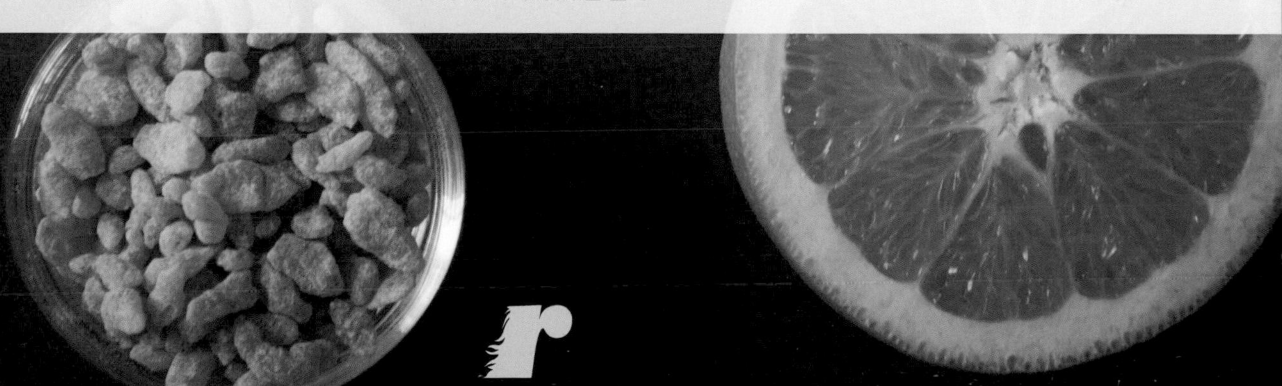

Racehorse Publishing

Racehorse Publishing books may be purchased in bulk at special discounts for sales promotion, corporate gifts, fund-raising, or educational purposes. Special editions can also be created to specifications. For details, contact the Special Sales Department, Skyhorse Publishing, 307 West 36th Street, 11th Floor, New York, NY 10018 or info@skyhorsepublishing.com.

Racehorse Publishing™ is a pending trademark of Skyhorse Publishing, Inc.®, a Delaware corporation.

Visit our website at www.skyhorsepublishing.com.

10 9 8 7 6 5 4 3 2

Library of Congress Cataloging-in-Publication Data is available on file.

Cover and interior photography by Brooke Lumbus Photography
Cover design by Michael Short
Additional photos by Pixabay

Print ISBN: 978-1-63158-587-6
eBook ISBN: 978-1-63158-270-7

Printed in China

Disclaimer

The information in this book is not intended to treat, cure, diagnose, or otherwise address medical conditions or ailments. This book is for educational, entertainment, and informational purposes only.

The contents of this book have been thoroughly reviewed for accuracy. However, the author and publisher disclaim any liability for any damages, losses, or injuries that may result from the use or misuse of any product or information presented herein. It is the purchaser's responsibility to read and follow all instructions and warnings on all product labels.

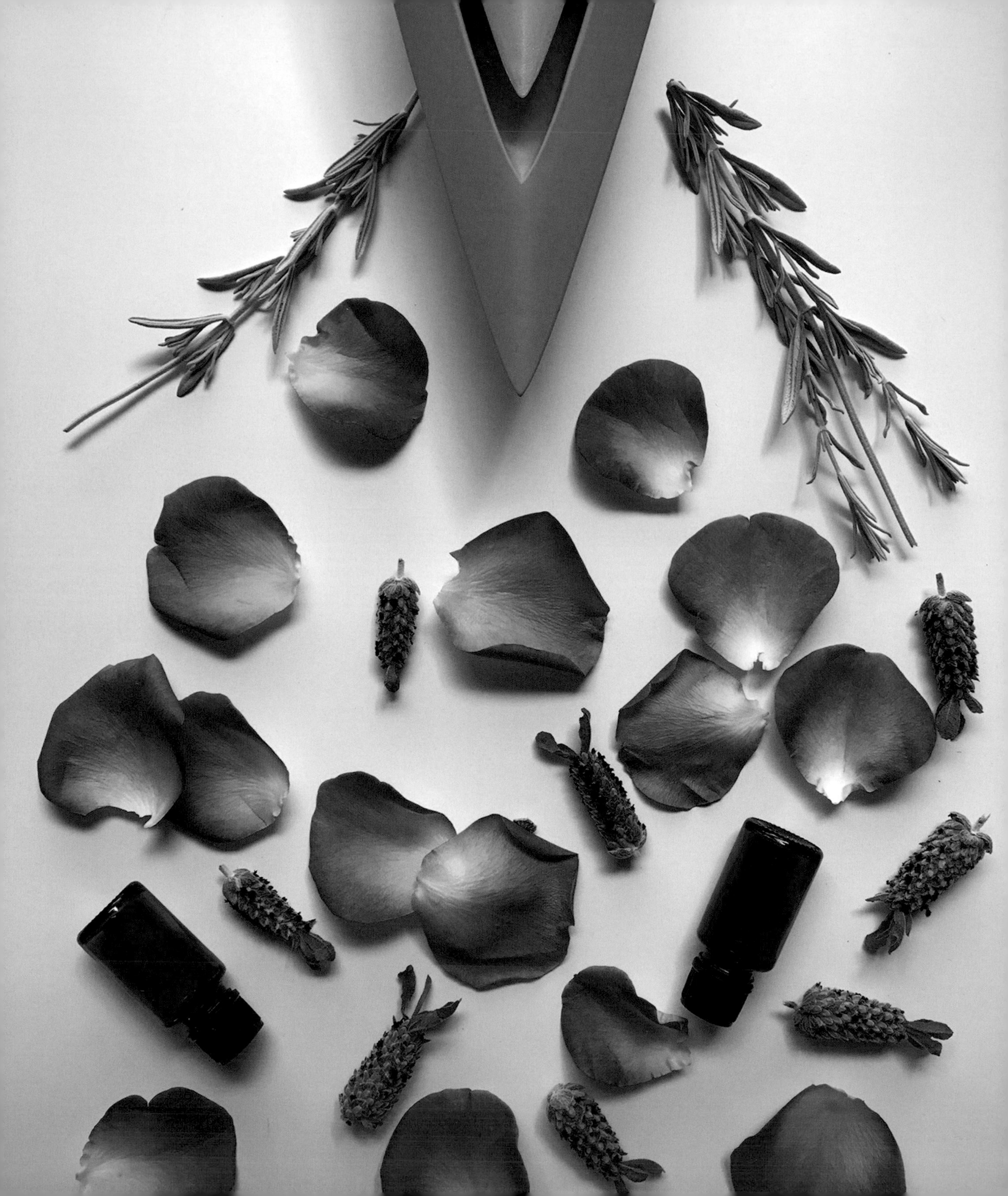

CONTENTS

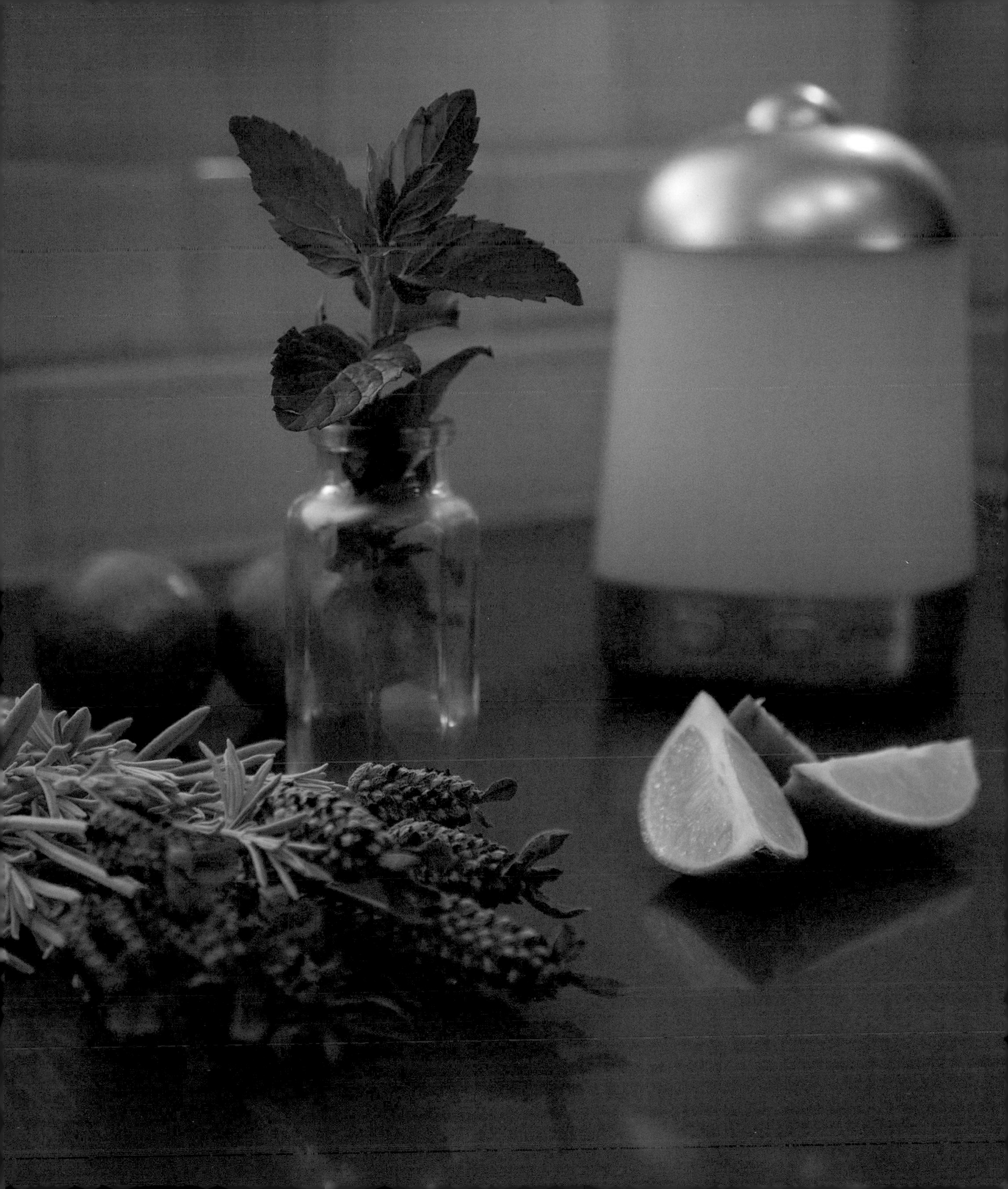

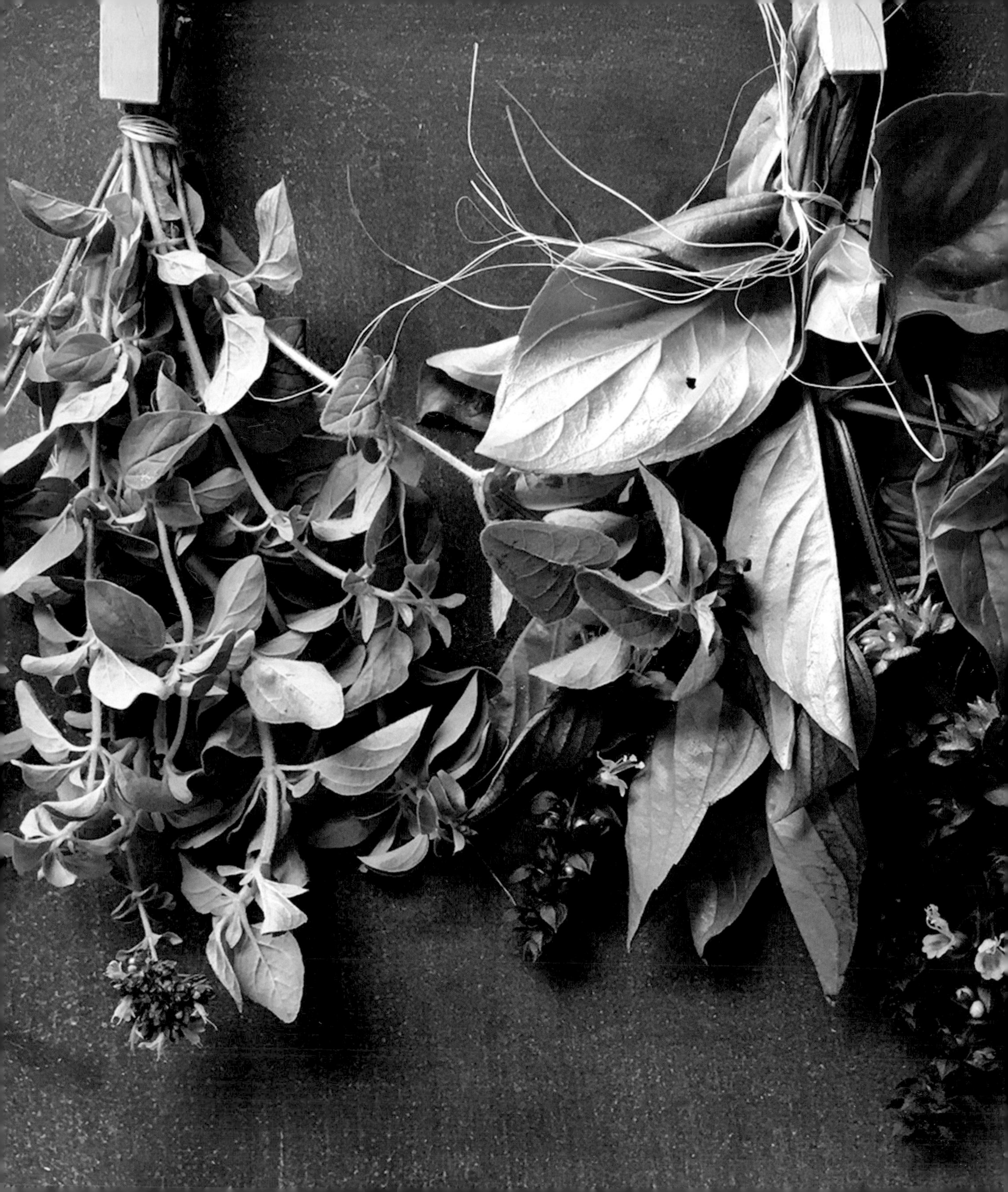

1
Why Diffuse Essential Oils?

What are essential oils?

Essential oils are naturally occurring compounds found in the seeds, roots, flowers, and other parts of plants. They are highly concentrated when distilled for purity and potency, and have been used for thousands of years for health, mood, and home.

Why diffuse essential oils?

Many of us grew up using air freshener sprays, gels, and plug-ins in our homes. What we didn't know then (but are learning now) is that many air fresheners use carcinogens—chemicals that can aggravate asthma and affect reproductive development.

Independent lab testing of spray, gel, and plug-in air fresheners confirmed the presence of phthalates (hormone-disrupting chemicals that could be a health risk to babies and young children) in 85 percent of products tested—including those marked "all natural." None of the products had these chemicals listed on their labels. (Source: nrdc.org/media/2007/070919)

"But wait!" you might say. "The ingredient list on my air freshener bottle says, 'Contains water, alcohol, odor eliminator derived from corn, fragrance.' Why aren't all those chemicals listed?"

For one single reason—they don't have to be.

Under the United States Federal Hazardous Substances Act (FHSA), manufacturers are not required to list all ingredients of household cleaners. This is ostensibly to protect their formulations from competitors—which is odd, because bread has all of its ingredients listed and there's no lack of competition in the bread aisle.

Pure, high-quality essential oils contain no fillers, artificial ingredients, pesticides, or other contaminants. That's why they are my choice for freshening the air and providing other health benefits. We have a diffuser in nearly every room of our home!

2
Quality is Critical

As with many products, essential oils are made in different grades or levels of quality.

- Synthetic oils or fragrance oils are the lowest quality and are typically used in lotions or perfumes. These are often sold at craft or health food stores.
- Food grade oils are used to flavor things like cake mix, cereal, etc. An example of this is the lemon or orange flavoring sold at the grocery store.
- Therapeutic grade oils are the highest grade and can be used aromatically (spread via air), topically (on the skin), or internally. I only use and recommend therapeutic grade oils, which you can learn more about at www.BrownThumbMama.com/oils.

There is no governing body regulating the quality of essential oils, so companies can make claims like "100 percent pure" or "natural" with few repercussions. There is no guarantee that these oils are pure. They may contain pesticide residues, solvents, contaminants, or synthetic compounds (which are much cheaper to produce).

Therapeutic grade essential oils are tested by independent laboratories to ensure they are completely pure and free of synthetics, contaminants, and pesticide residues. After meeting these stringent requirements, they are labeled safe by the Food & Drug Administration (FDA) for topical or internal use.

3
A Word About Safety

Essential oils are highly potent plant extracts and should be used with care. They are safe and effective when used correctly, and it only takes a small amount to see powerful therapeutic benefits. Remember:

- Never apply essential oils directly to the eyes, the ears, the nose, or other sensitive areas. To dilute essential oils, apply coconut oil or another vegetable oil (not water).
- It's important to use only therapeutic quality essential oils, read all labels thoroughly, and use common sense.
- Essential oil diffusers are electrical appliances and should not be used around water.

Parents: Therapeutic quality oils are safe to use with children when highly diluted. When diffusing oils in a child's room, reduce the number of drops in the recipe and diffuse for a few minutes at a time.

Pet Owners: An animal's sense of smell is so much more powerful than our own. Because of this, they must be able to leave the room if a smell becomes overwhelming to them. Do not diffuse essential oils in a closed room that the animal cannot leave.

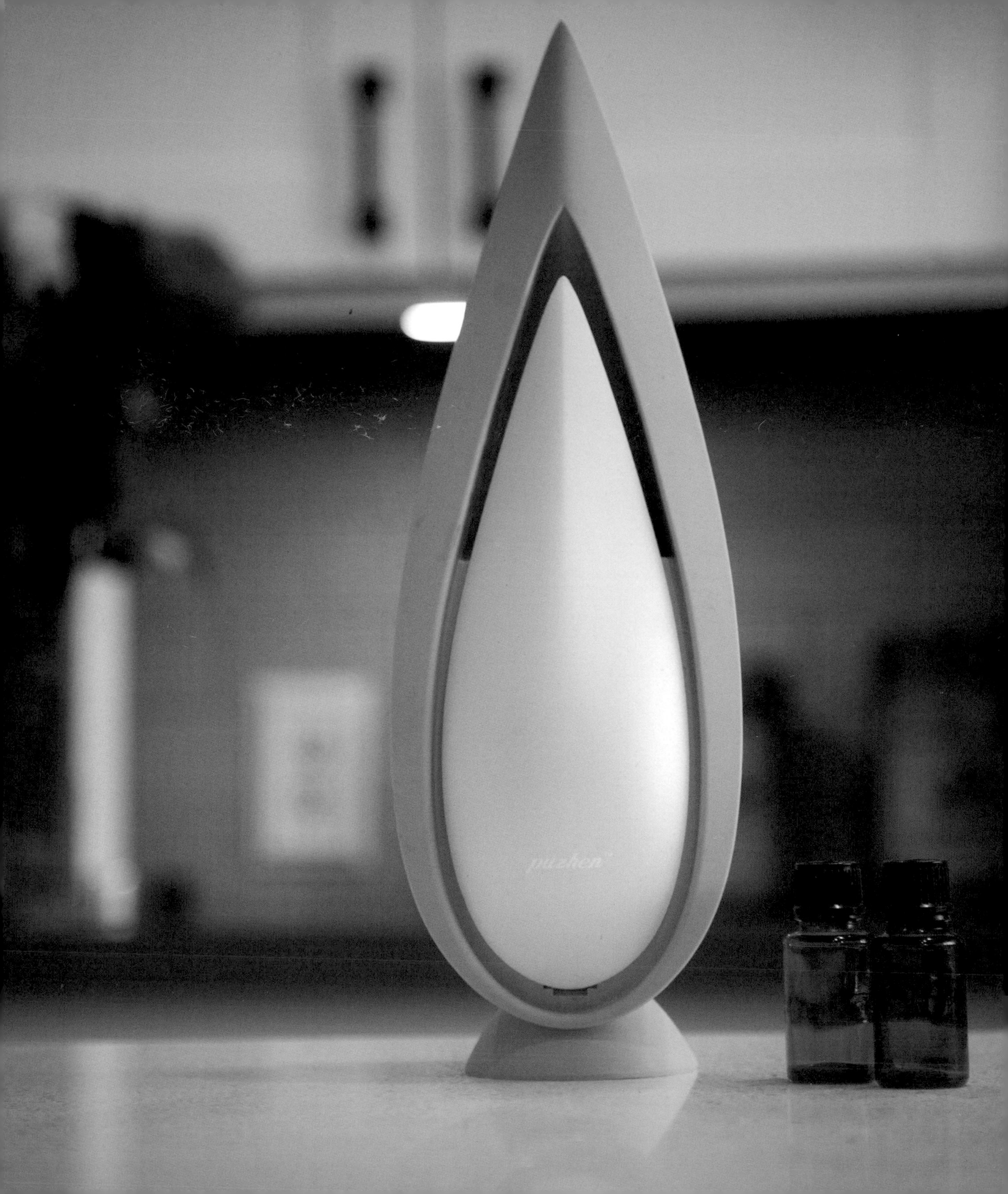
puzhen

4
Types of Diffusers

There are two main types of essential oil diffusers: ultrasonic and nebulizing. The primary difference is that ultrasonic diffusers use water and nebulizing diffusers do not.

Ultrasonic diffusers agitate water and essential oils at millions of vibrations per second. This converts the water into a fine mist and converts the oil into micro-particles that are released into the air. The mist emitted is so fine that if you hold your hand over the diffuser, your hand doesn't get wet.

Nebulizing diffusers pressurize air and draw oils through a special nozzle. This breaks the oils down into minute particles and disperses them into the air in short bursts. These diffusers don't use water, but can use an entire bottle of oil quickly if diffuser settings are not correct.

It's important to compare the features of the different types of diffusers before you make a purchase. Here are some important pros and cons about both ultrasonic and nebulizing diffusers.

	Ultrasonic	Nebulizing
Water	Yes	No
Cost	Less expensive	More expensive
Light	Often included	No
Oil Concentration	Lower	Higher
Cleaning	Occasionally	Never
Sound	Quiet	Louder

Heat diffusers are not a good idea because they change the chemical properties of the oils. Don't burn essential oils in a wax burner or similar contraption.

How Long to Diffuse

Most quality diffusers will turn off after a certain amount of time, or when the reservoir empties. You don't need to diffuse continuously to get benefits from the oils! Here are some tips to get you started:

- Run your diffuser between thirty minutes to an hour to freshen a room.
- Diffuse for one to two hours at bedtime to help kids fall asleep.
- To promote restful sleep, diffuse the Breathe Easy essential oil combination all night.

5

How to Clean Your Diffuser

Most diffusers come with cleaning instructions, but heaven knows that we don't always keep those little booklets handy.

Keeping your diffuser clean will enhance its performance and keep it running longer. It's easy to clean your diffuser, and no special ingredients or tools are needed.

Unplug the diffuser and empty out any residual liquid in it. Fill the diffuser reservoir halfway with tap water and halfway with plain white vinegar.

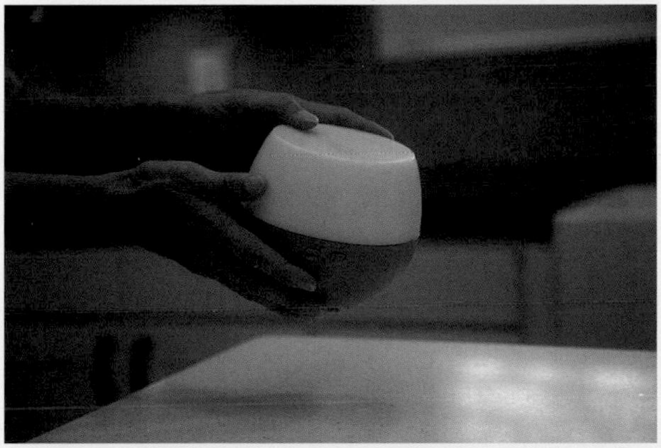

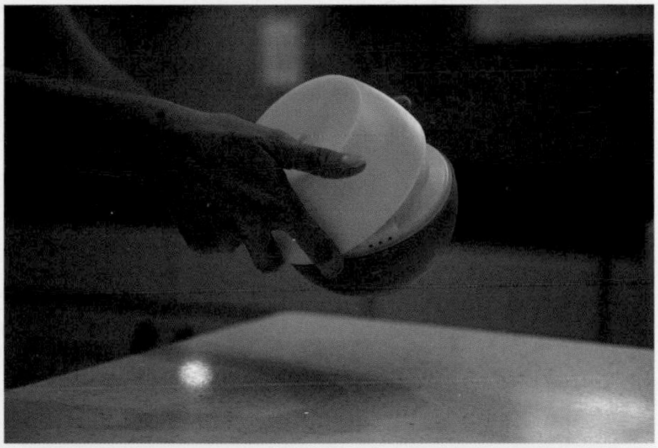

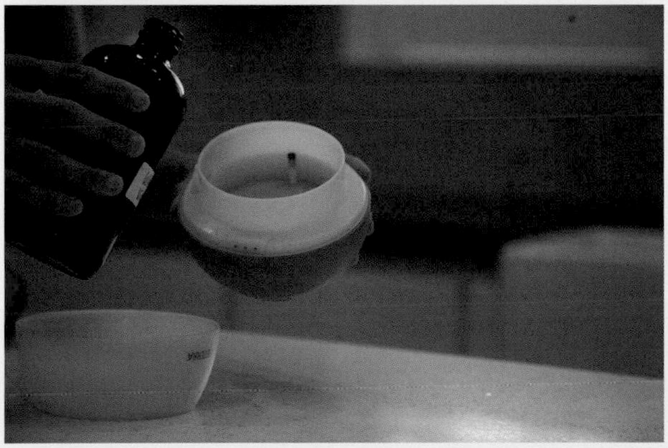

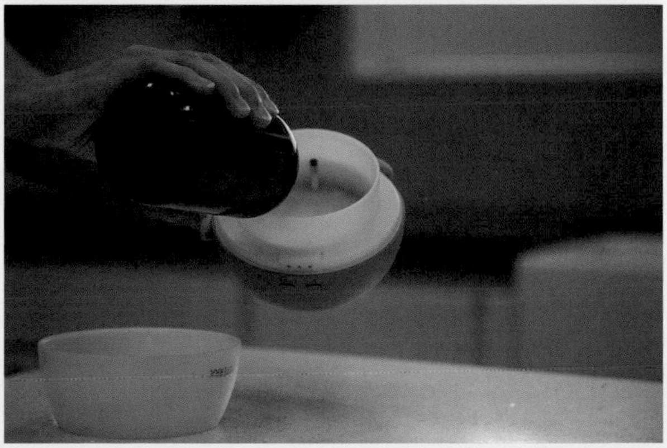

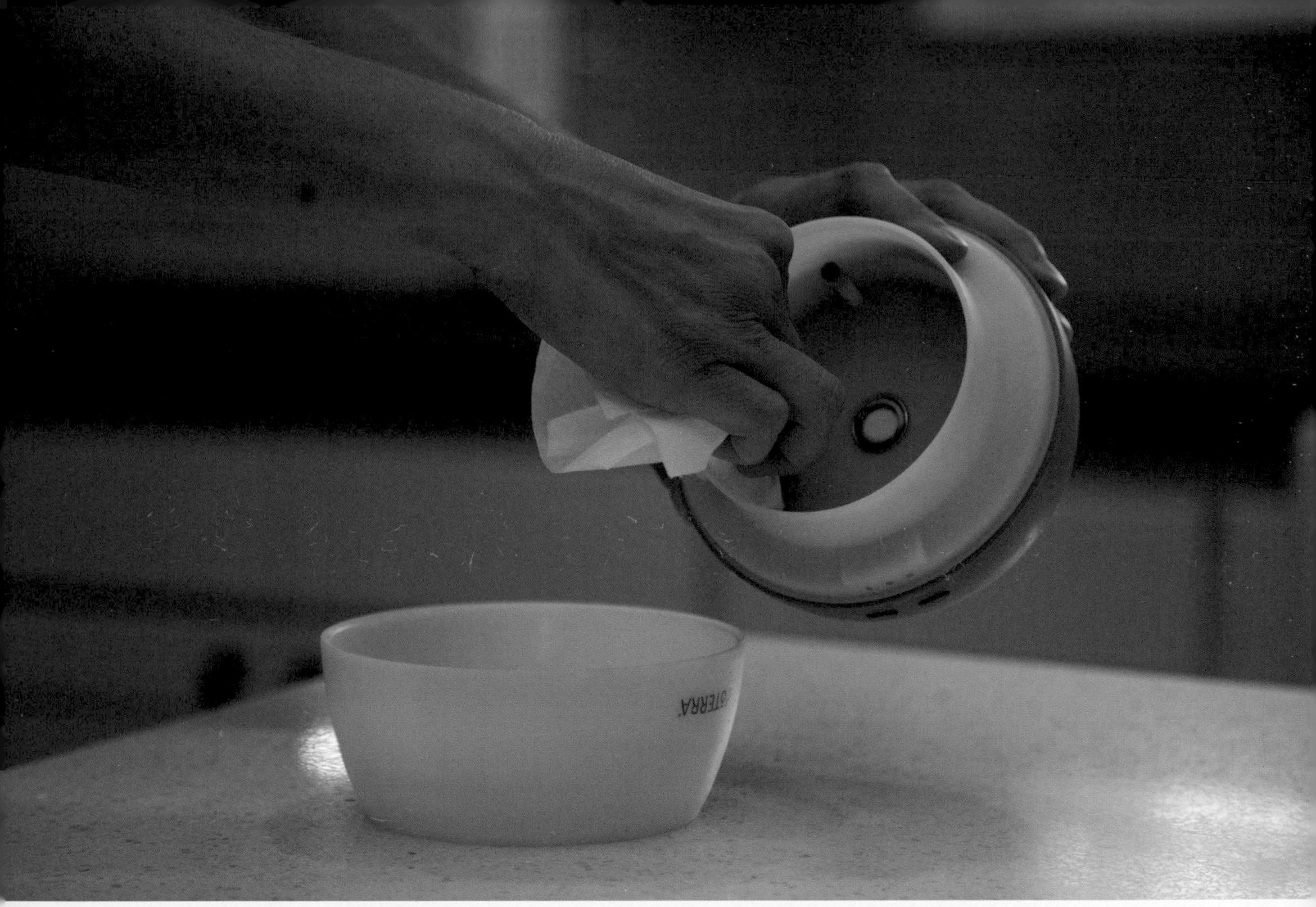

Run it for a few minutes and then carefully pour out any leftover liquid. (Note: If water gets into the motor or the inside of the housing, the diffuser will be ruined.)

Use a paper towel or cotton cloth to wipe any deposits from the corners or tight spots. Be sure to clean the sensor, since that's a critical part of the machine. Wipe the outside dry with a clean cloth and you're done.

Clean your diffuser at least once a month to remove any buildup of smells or hard water.

6
Diffuser Recipes

Ultrasonic diffusers use different amounts of water, depending on the model. Most are from 70mL to 150mL (5–10 tablespoons). These recipes are made for a 70mL diffuser, so they can easily be doubled.

If you have a nebulizing diffuser, you can still use these recipes. Mix the oils in the proportions specified in an empty oil bottle and label it with the name of the blend. Then attach the bottle to your nebulizer as usual.

Note: Each diffuser recipe title has five little drops below the name so you can remember how you and your family like it. Score each recipe from one drop (not so great) to five drops (loved it!).

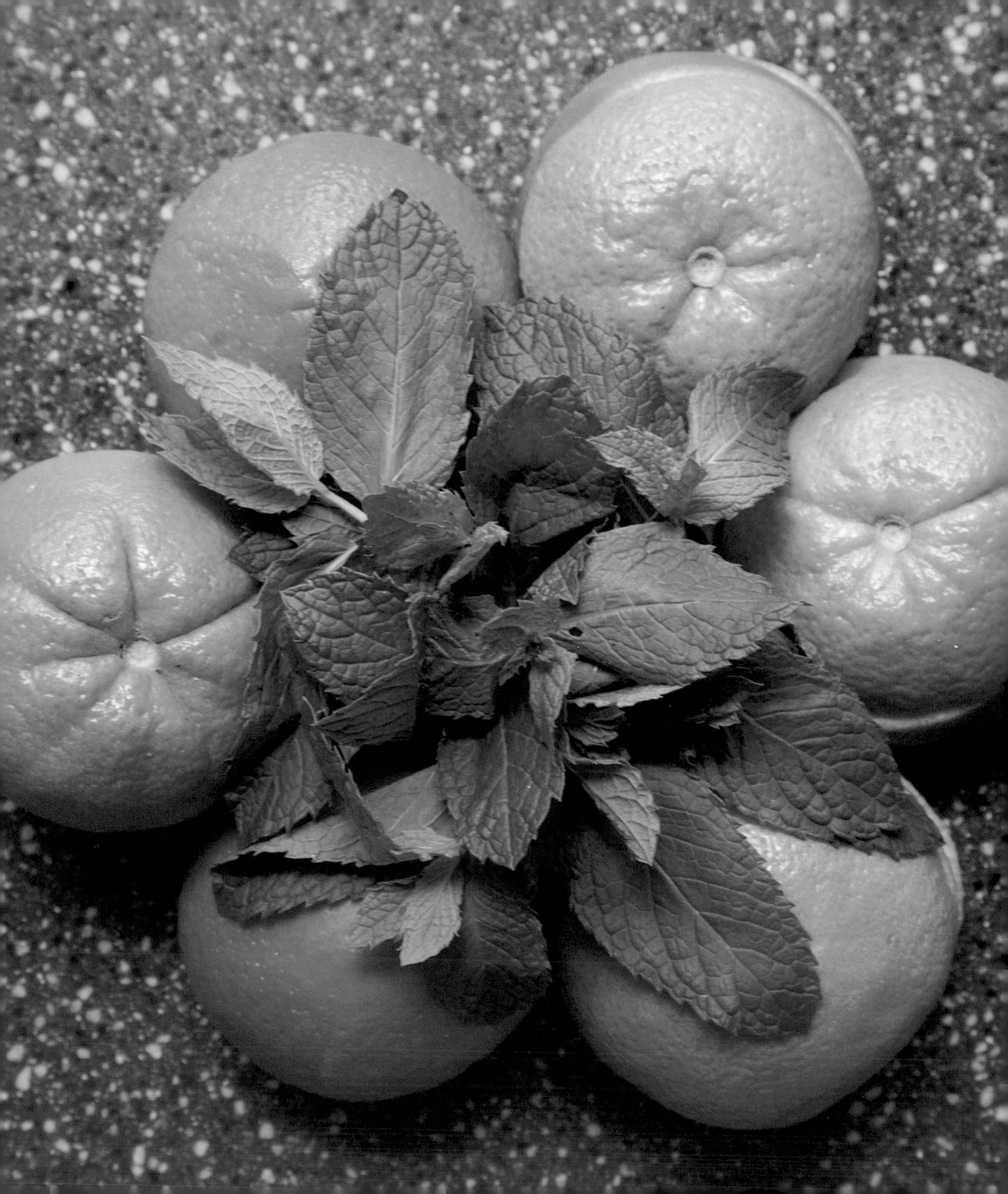

7

Energizing

Skip the coffee and energy drinks and enjoy a natural boost with these diffuser blends. They're a great way to start the day or to spark your energy during the afternoon slump.

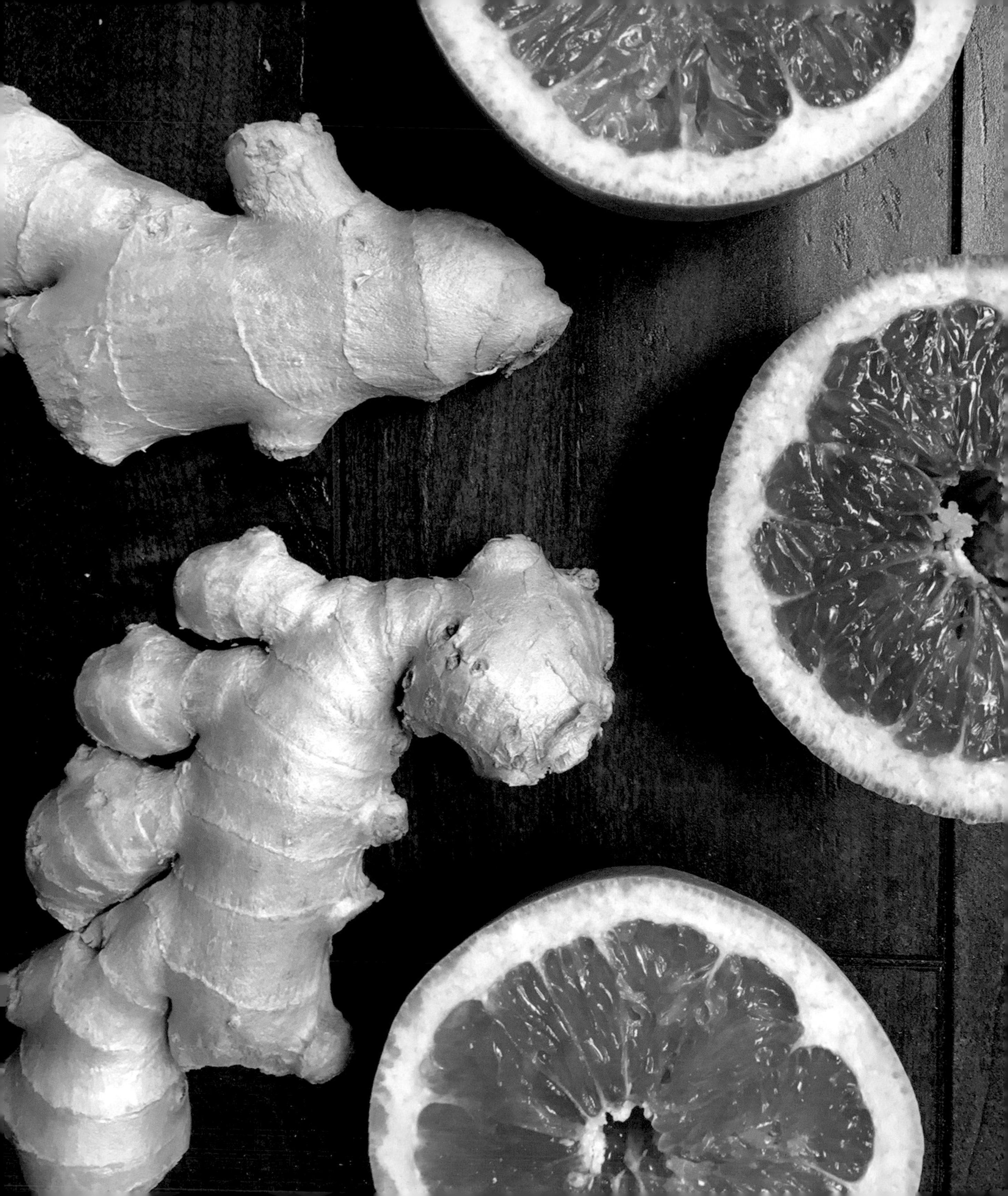

Wake Me Up

- 2 drops Peppermint essential oil
- 2 drops Wild Orange essential oil

Bright and Fresh

- 3 drops Tangerine essential oil
- 2 drops Bergamot essential oil
- 1 drop Douglas Fir essential oil

Mama's Little Helper

- 2 drops Ginger essential oil
- 3 drops Grapefruit essential oil

Pep in Your Step

- 2 drops Basil essential oil
- 2 drops Grapefruit essential oil
- 1 drop Cypress essential oil

Elevate Me

- 4 drops Lime essential oil
- 2 drops Spearmint essential oil
- 1 drop Red Mandarin essential oil

Motivation

- 3 drops Peppermint essential oil
- 3 drops Rosemary essential oil
- 2 drops Grapefruit essential oil

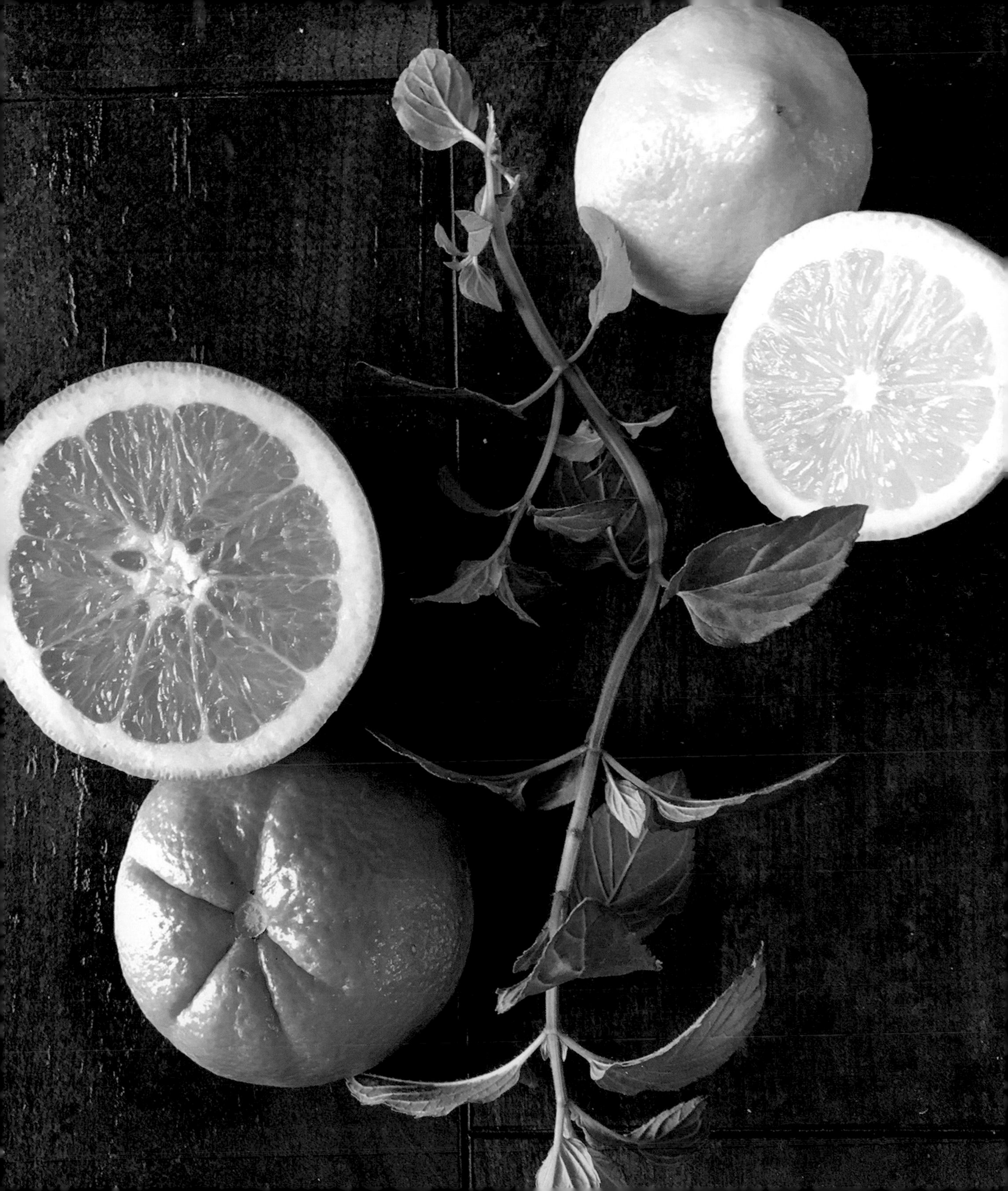

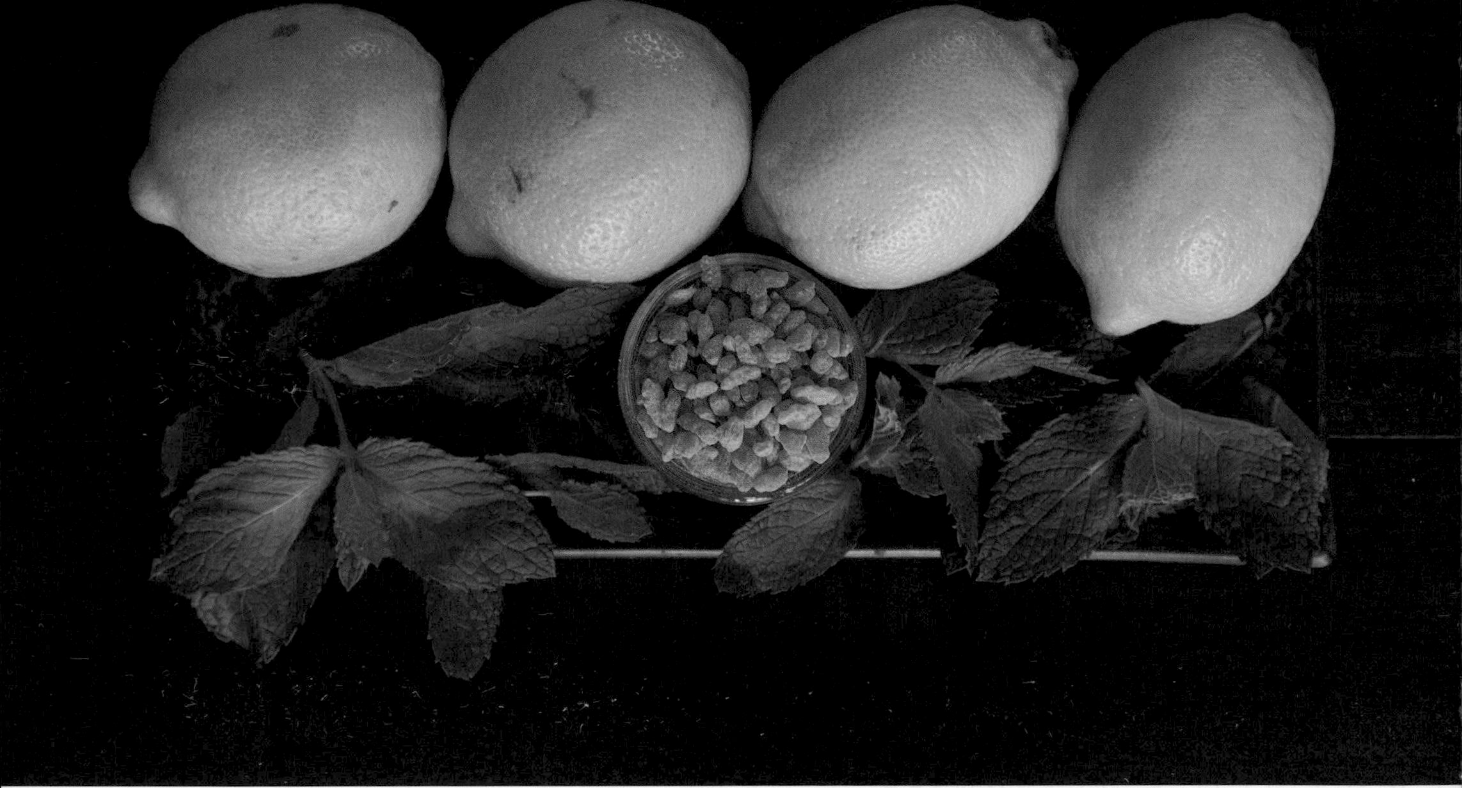

Power Hour

- 2 drops Lemon essential oil
- 2 drops Peppermint essential oil
- 1 drop Frankincense essential oil

Good Day Sunshine

- 2 drops Cinnamon essential oil
- 2 drops Frankincense essential oil
- 2 drops Wild Orange essential oil

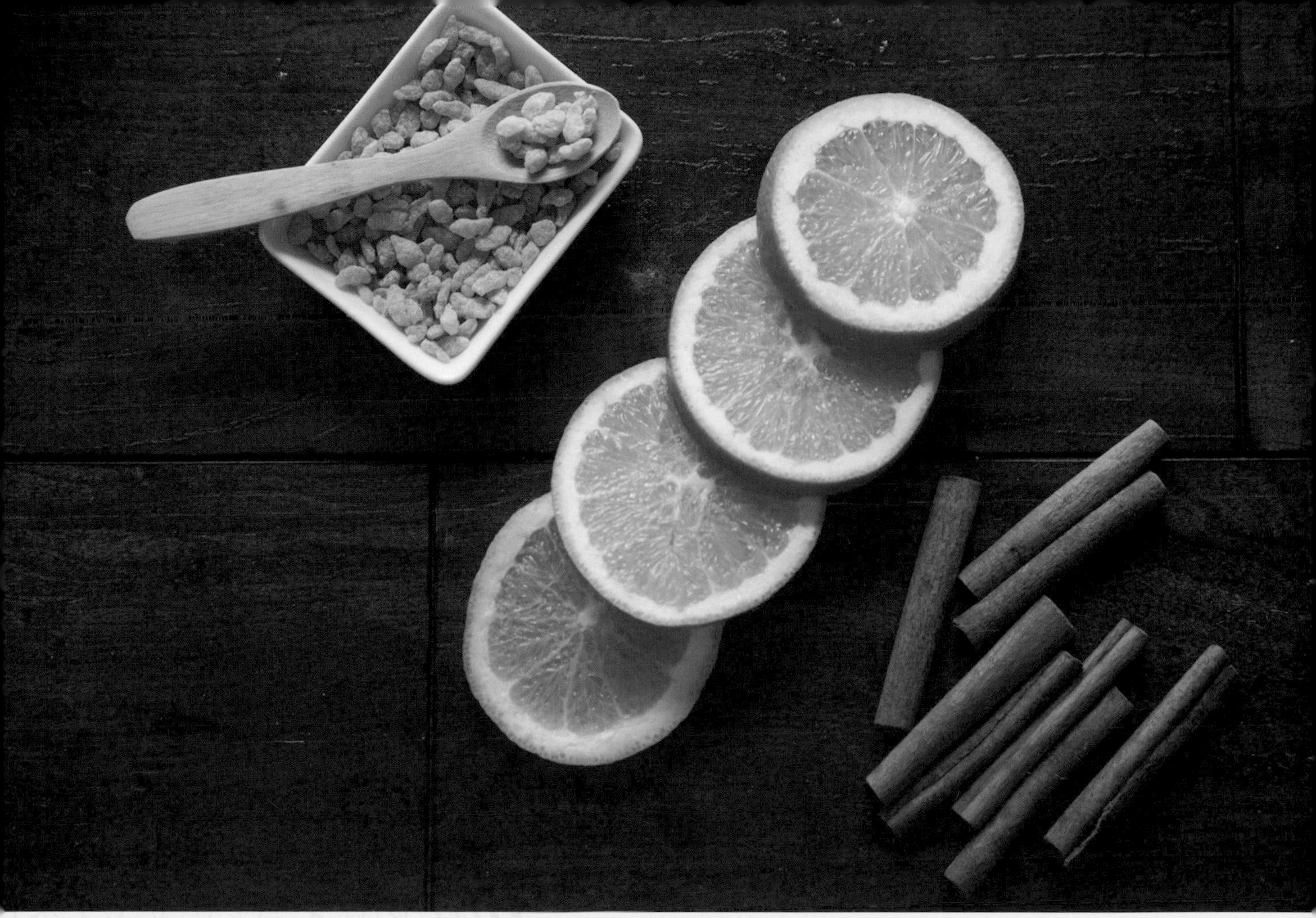

Welcome to My Morning

- 1 drop Basil essential oil
- 1 drop Clove essential oil
- 1 drop Lemon essential oil
- 1 drop Peppermint essential oil
- 1 drop Wild Orange essential oil

8

Mental Clarity

Whether you're prepping for a big meeting, settling the kids down for homework time, or doing anything else where focus is needed, these recipes are for you.

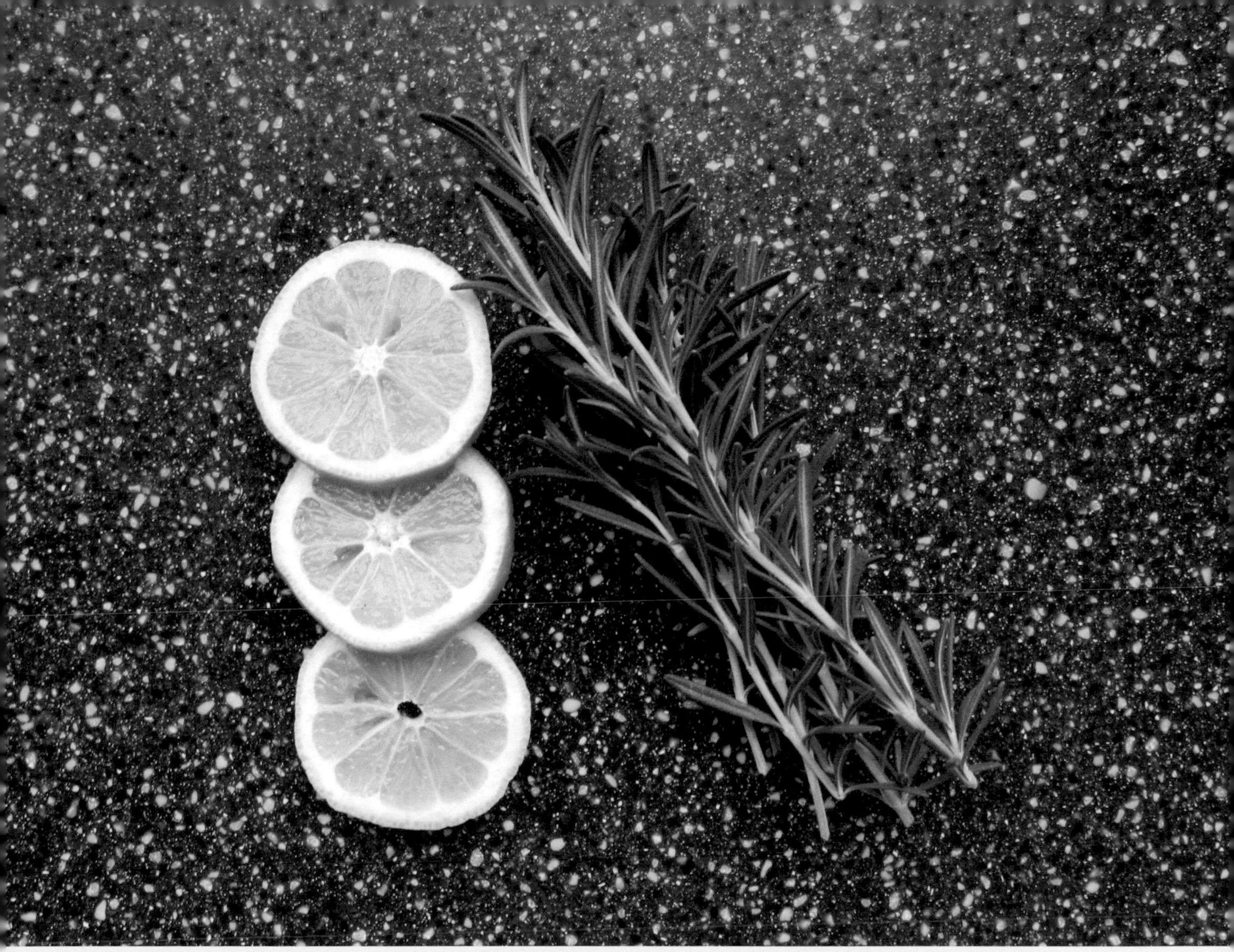

On Point

- 2 drops Lemon essential oil
- 3 drops Rosemary essential oil

Sharp as a Tack

- 4 drops Cypress essential oil
- 1 drop Peppermint essential oil

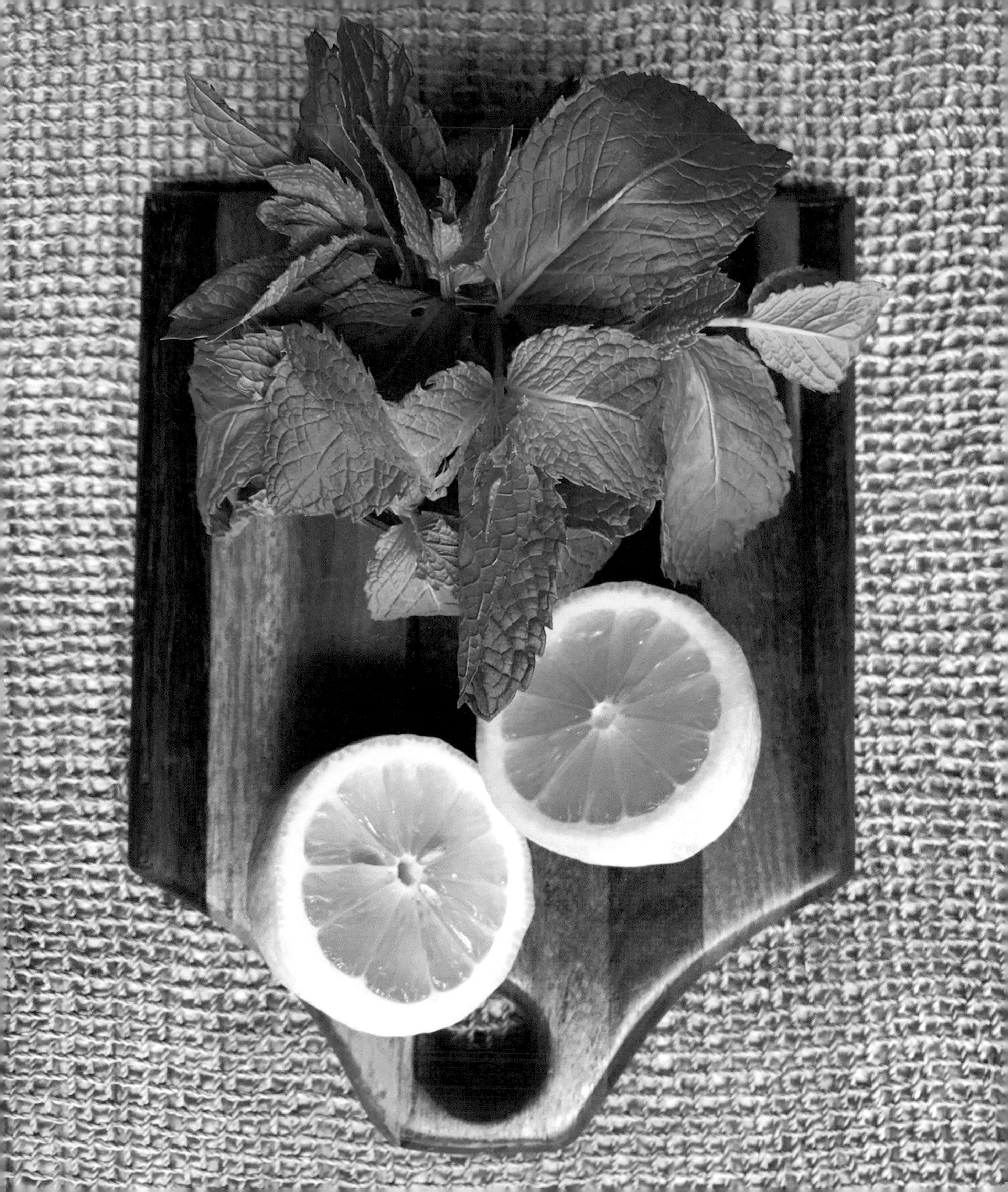

Freshly Focused

- 3 drops Lemon essential oil
- 2 drops Peppermint essential oil

Clarity

- 3 drops Bergamot essential oil
- 2 drops Rosemary essential oil

Pure Concentration

- 2 drops Cypress essential oil
- 2 drops Rosemary essential oil
- 1 drop Basil essential oil

Smarty Pants

- 2 drops Clary Sage essential oil
- 2 drops Rosemary essential oil
- 2 drops Wild Orange essential oil

Laser Focus

- 2 drops Frankincense essential oil
- 1 drop Sandalwood essential oil
- 1 drop Cinnamon Bark essential oil

Zen Monk Mind

- 1 drop Clary Sage essential oil
- 1 drop Lavender essential oil
- 1 drop Sandalwood essential oil
- 1 drop Wild Orange essential oil

Break on Through

- 3 drops Grapefruit essential oil
- 2 drops Lime essential oil
- 1 drop Black Pepper essential oil
- 1 drop Peppermint essential oil
- 1 drop Rosemary essential oil

9

Lift Your Mood

Everyone has days when they're feeling low and need a little boost. These exotic and comforting smells will uplift and inspire you.

Renew

- 3 drops Bergamot essential oil
- 2 drops Clary Sage essential oil

Nature's Bliss

- 3 drops Bergamot essential oil
- 2 drops Patchouli essential oil

Rise and Shine

- 2 drops Lemon essential oil
- 2 drops Peppermint essential oil
- 2 drops Wild Orange essential oil

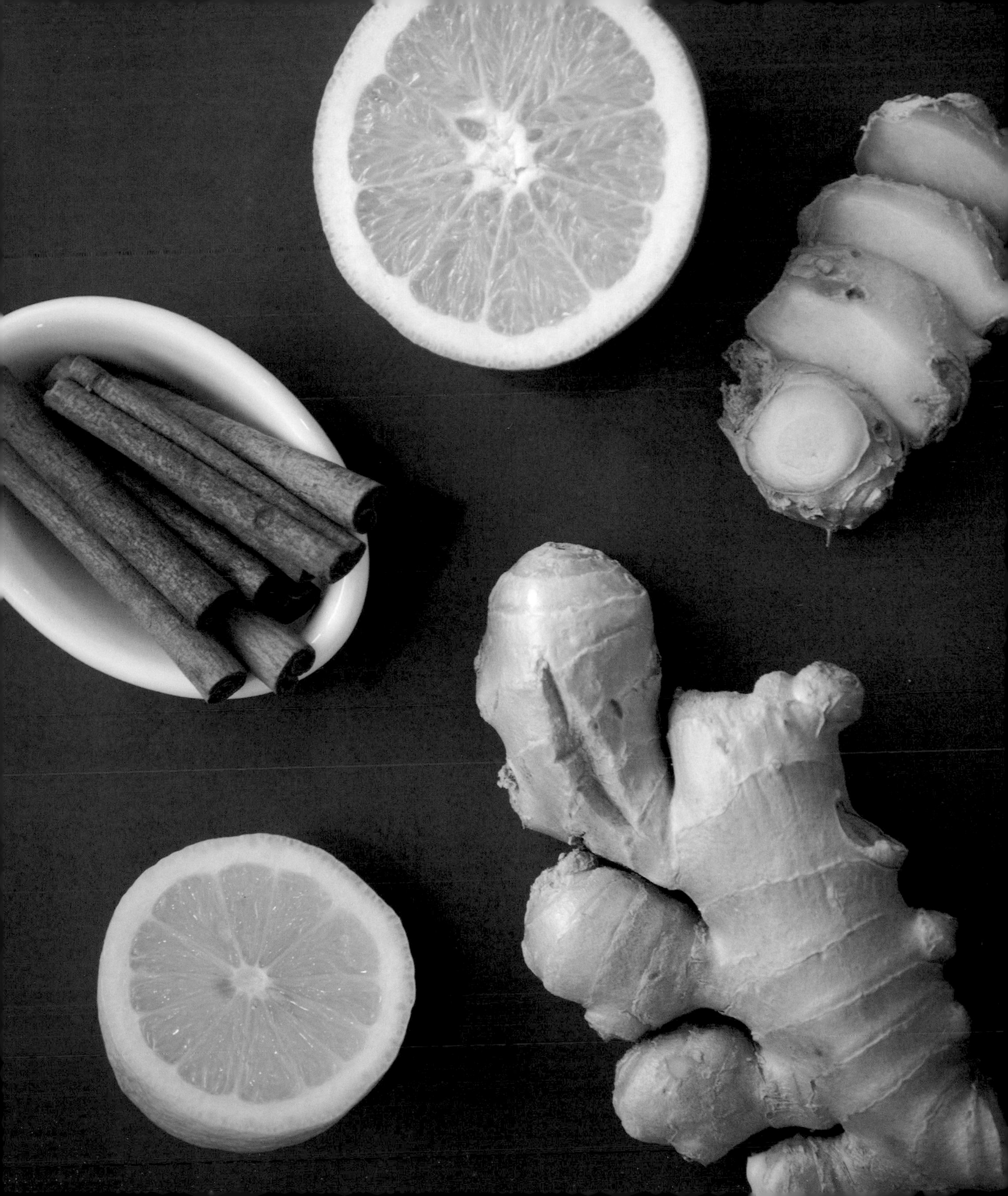

Inspire

- 2 drops Frankincense essential oil
- 2 drops Jasmine essential oil
- 1 drop Lemon essential oil

Fresh Start

- 2 drops Lemongrass essential oil
- 2 drops Spearmint essential oil
- 2 drops Tangerine essential oil

Esteem

- 3 drops Bergamot essential oil
- 3 drops Lavender essential oil
- 2 drops Geranium essential oil

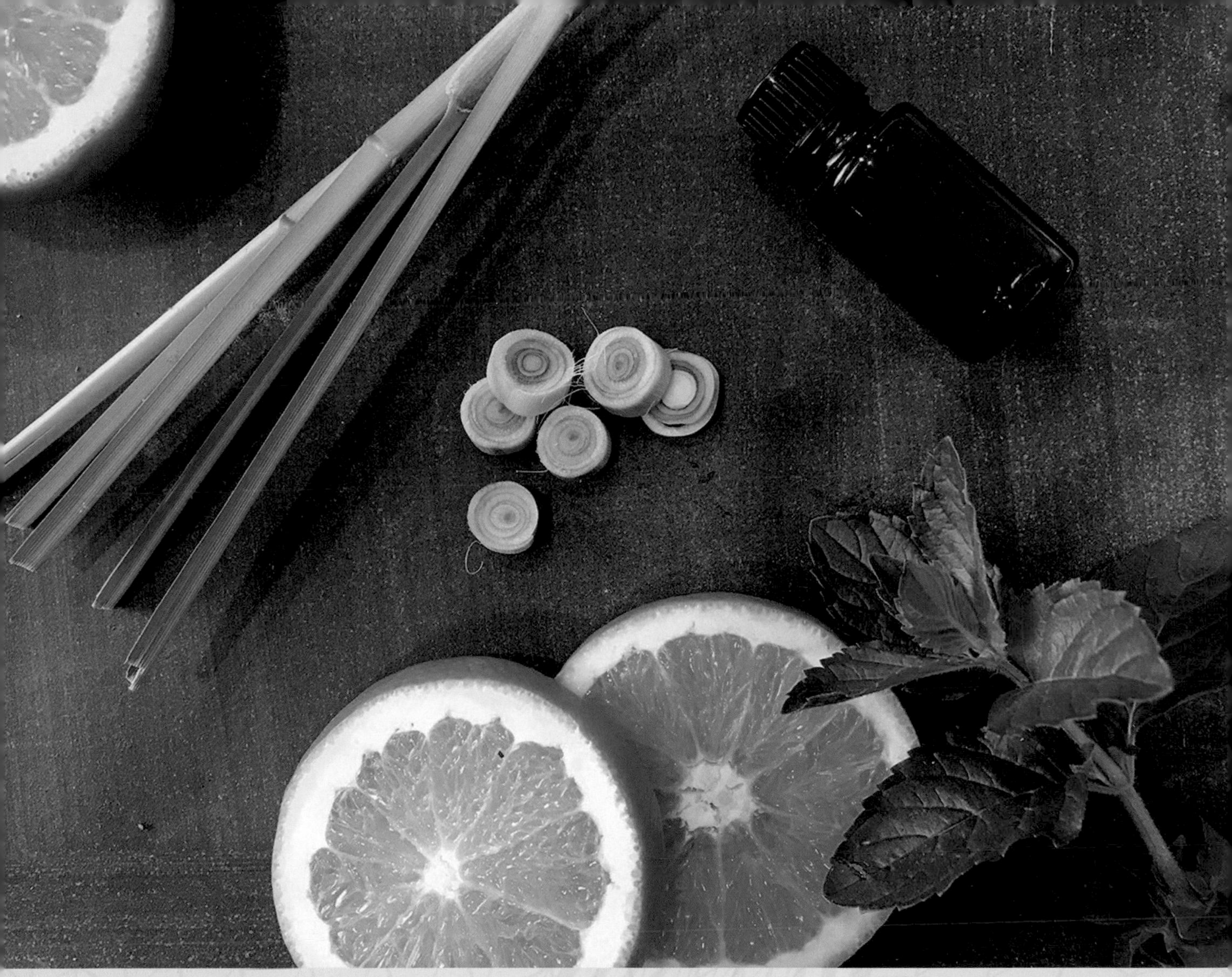

Sweet and Sassy

- 3 drops Bergamot essential oil
- 2 drops Geranium essential oil
- 1 drop Ginger essential oil

Refreshing

- 3 drops Grapefruit essential oil
- 2 drops Bergamot essential oil
- 1 drop Lavender essential oil
- 1 drop Ylang Ylang essential oil

Explore the Possibilities

- 2 drops Bergamot essential oil
- 2 drops Cypress essential oil
- 2 drops Frankincense essential oil
- 2 drops Wild Orange essential oil

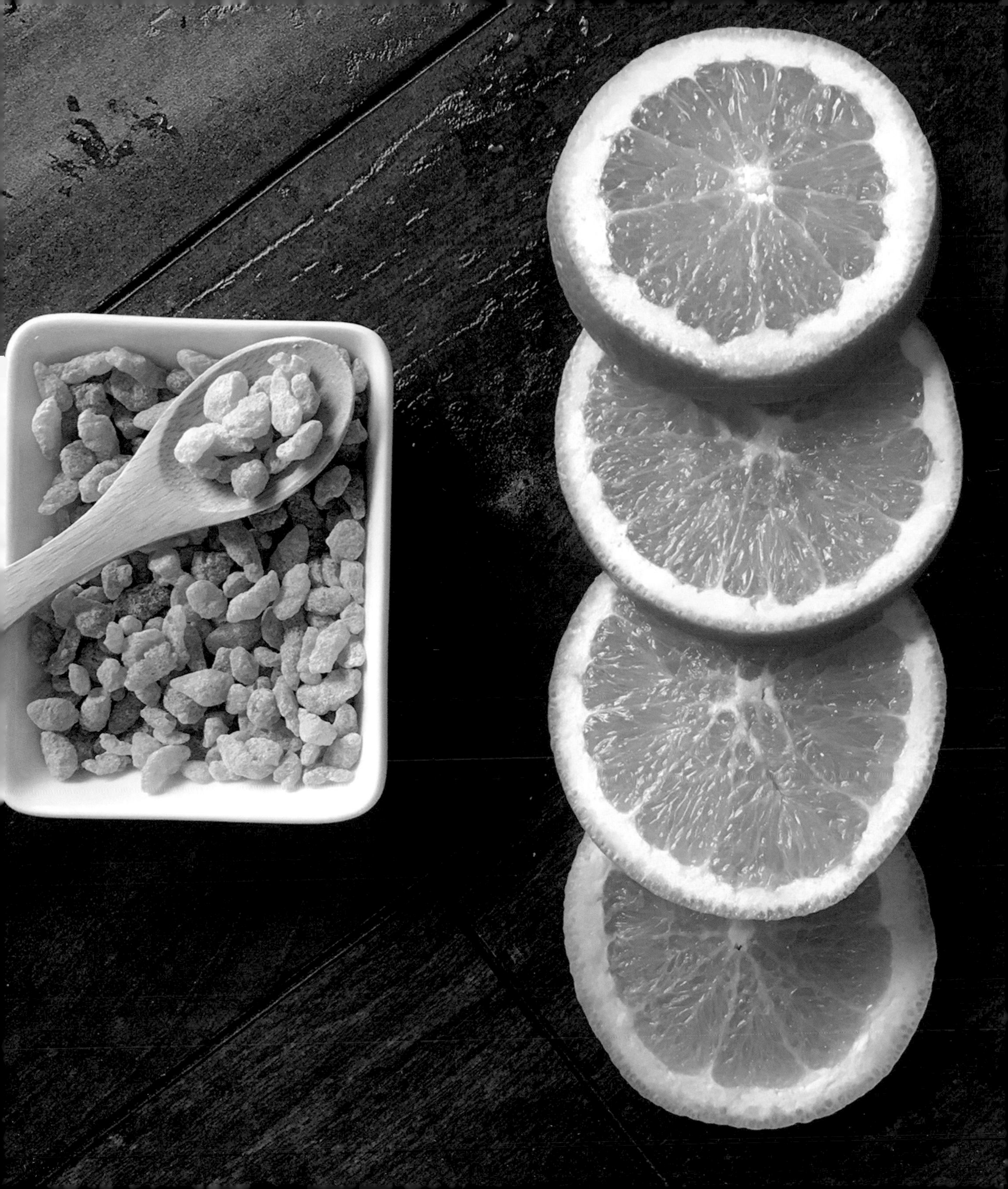

10

Around the House

Pure essential oils have many therapeutic benefits—and they're also great for purifying and freshening the air. These combinations will give your home a bright, clean scent.

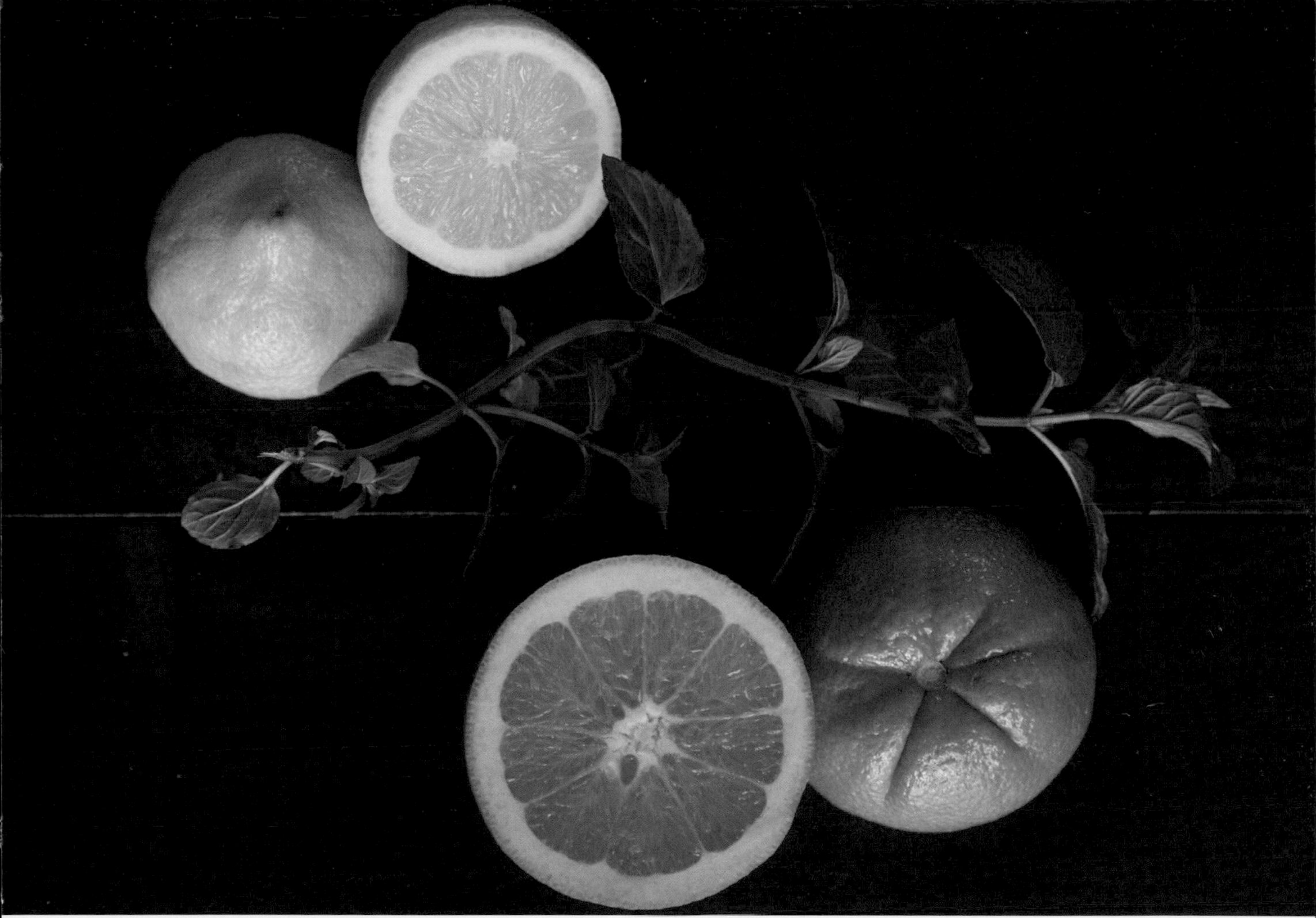

Sunny Day

- 3 drops Lemon essential oil
- 3 drops Tangerine essential oil
- 1 drop Spearmint essential oil

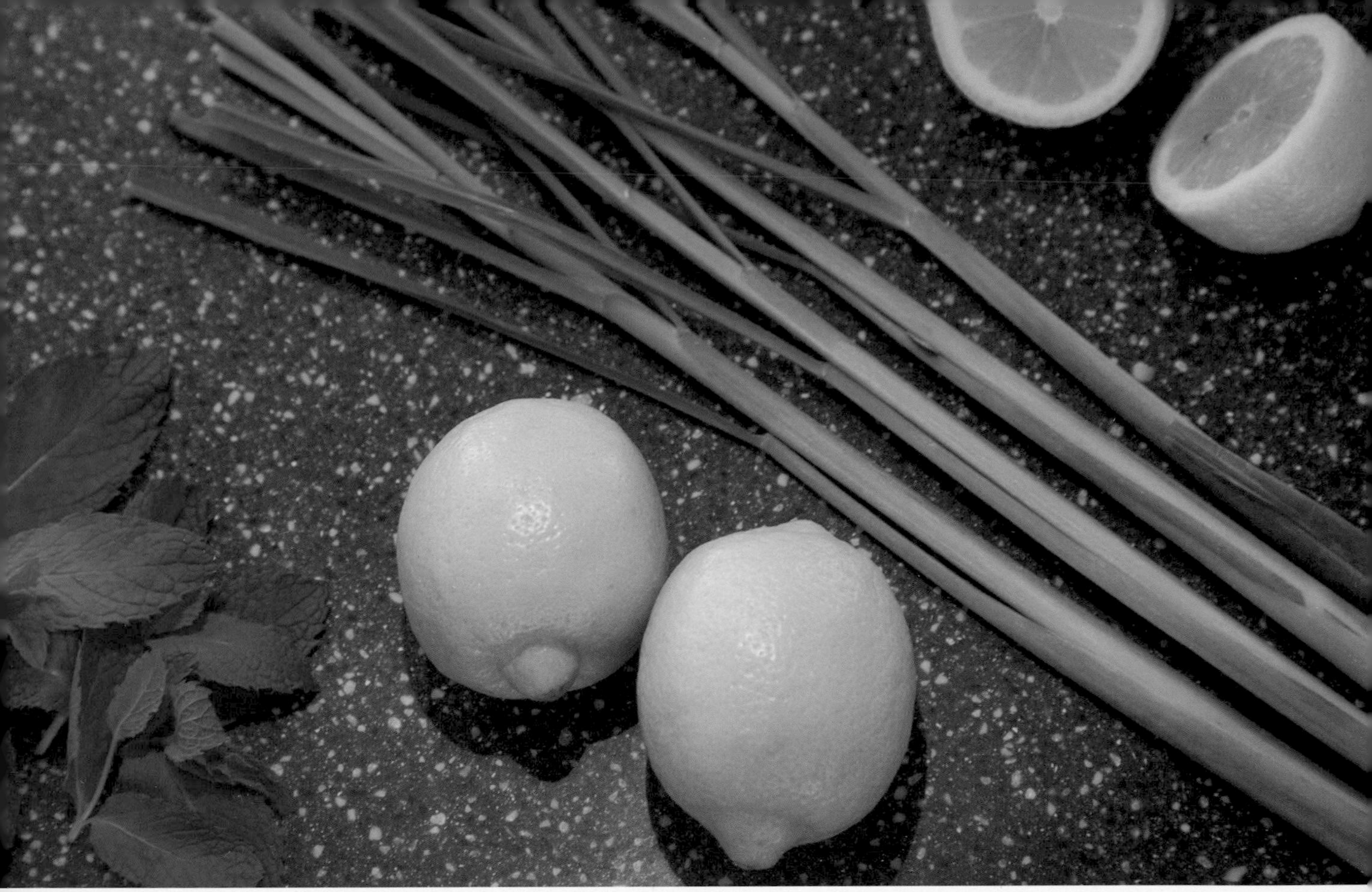

Refresh Mint

- 5 drops Lemon essential oil
- 4 drops Lemongrass essential oil
- 2 drops Peppermint essential oil

Almost Paradise

- 3 drops Lavender essential oil
- 2 drops Bergamot essential oil
- 1 drop Lemon essential oil
- 1 drop Sandalwood essential oil

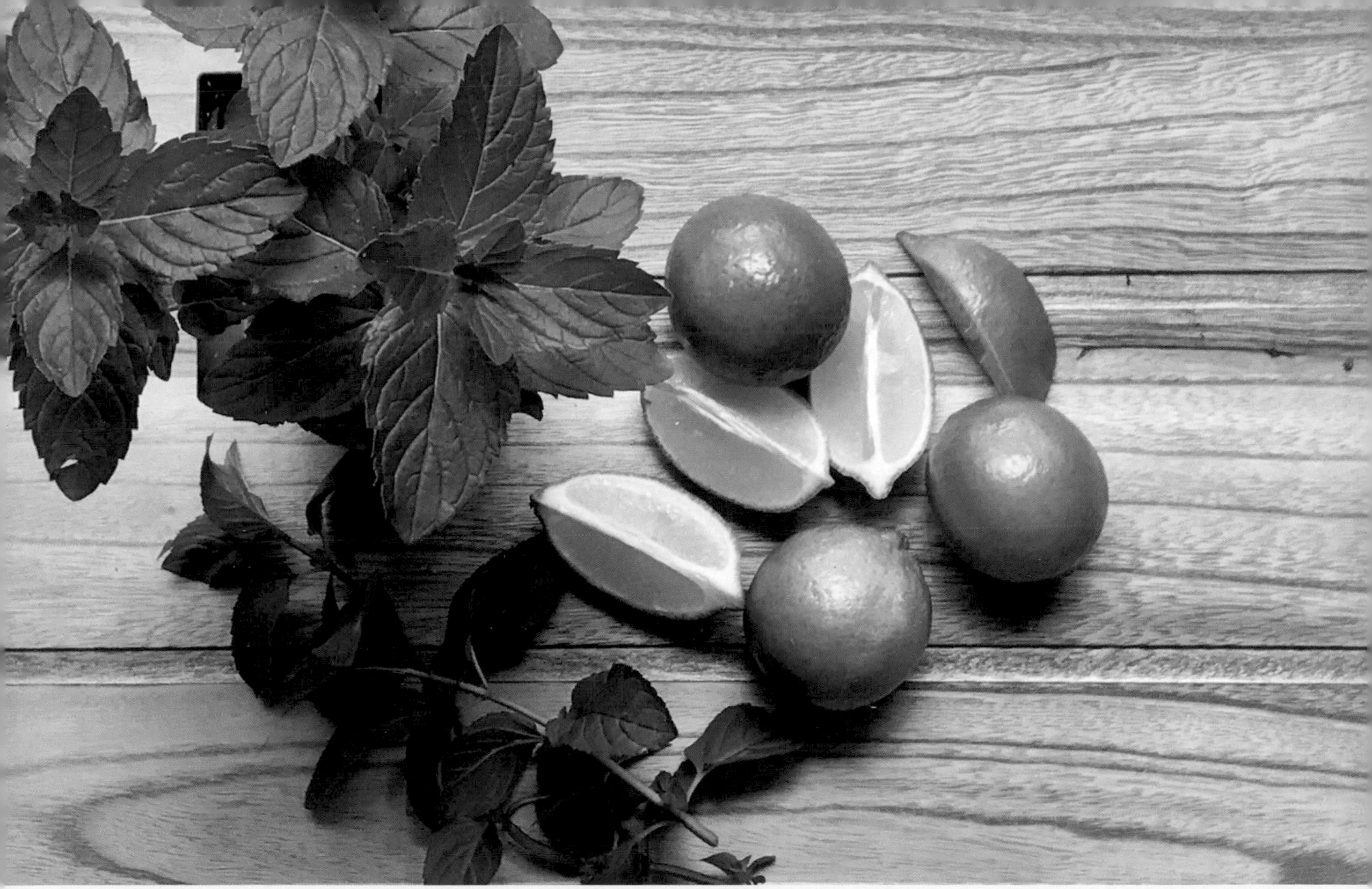

Spellbound

- 4 drops Eucalyptus essential oil
- 2 drops Cinnamon essential oil
- 2 drops Lemongrass essential oil

Margarita Sunrise

- 2 drops Grapefruit essential oil
- 2 drops Lime essential oil
- 2 drops Spearmint essential oil
- 2 drops Tangerine essential oil

Forest Staycation

- 2 drops Cedarwood essential oil
- 2 drops Lavender essential oil
- 2 drops Pine essential oil
- 2 drops Spearmint essential oil

Thyme to Uplift

- 3 drops Grapefruit essential oil
- 3 drops Lemon essential oil
- 3 drops Thyme essential oil

Tel Aviv

- 2 drops Cedarwood essential oil
- 2 drops Lavender essential oil
- 2 drops Melaleuca essential oil
- 2 drops Wild Orange essential oil

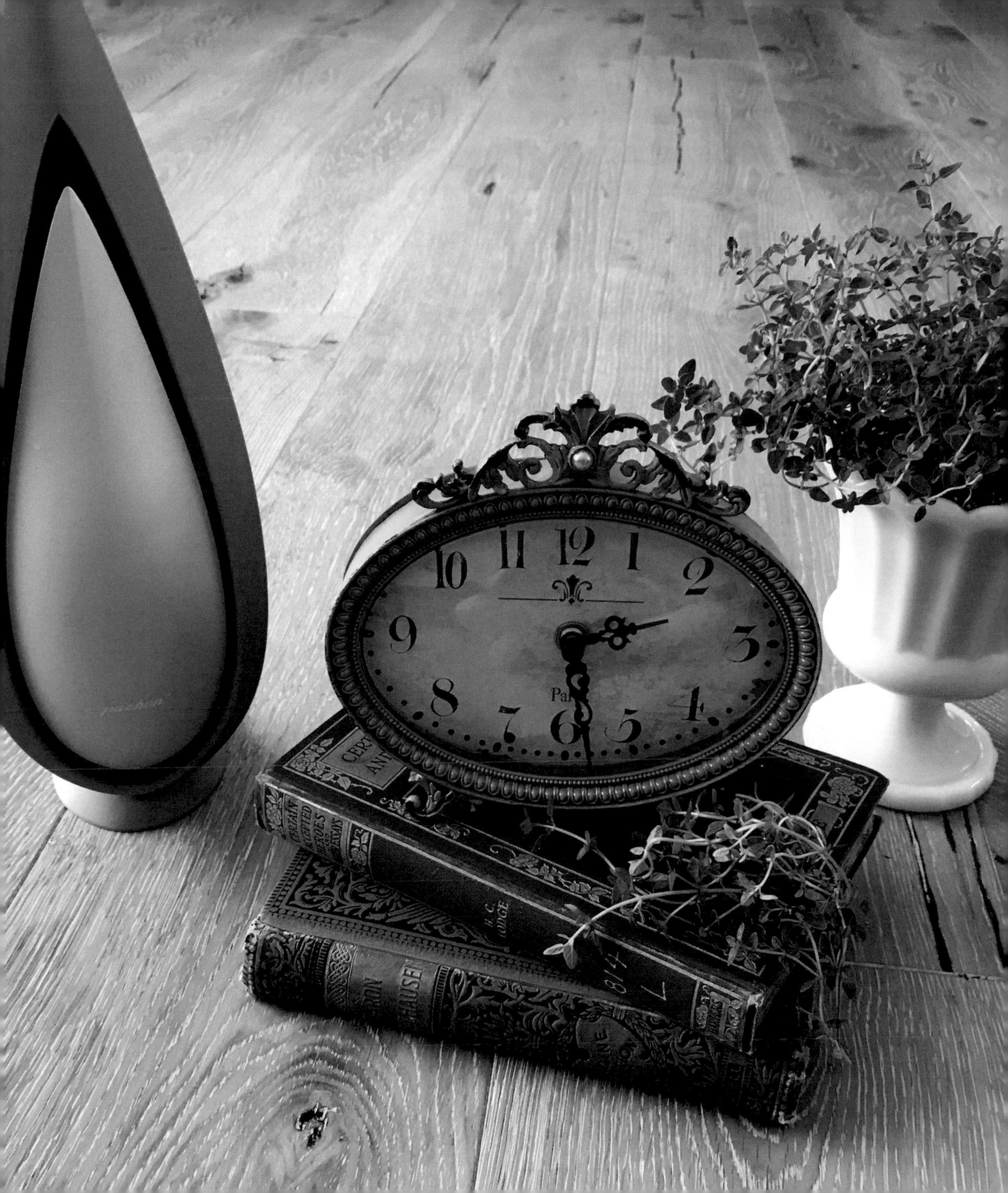

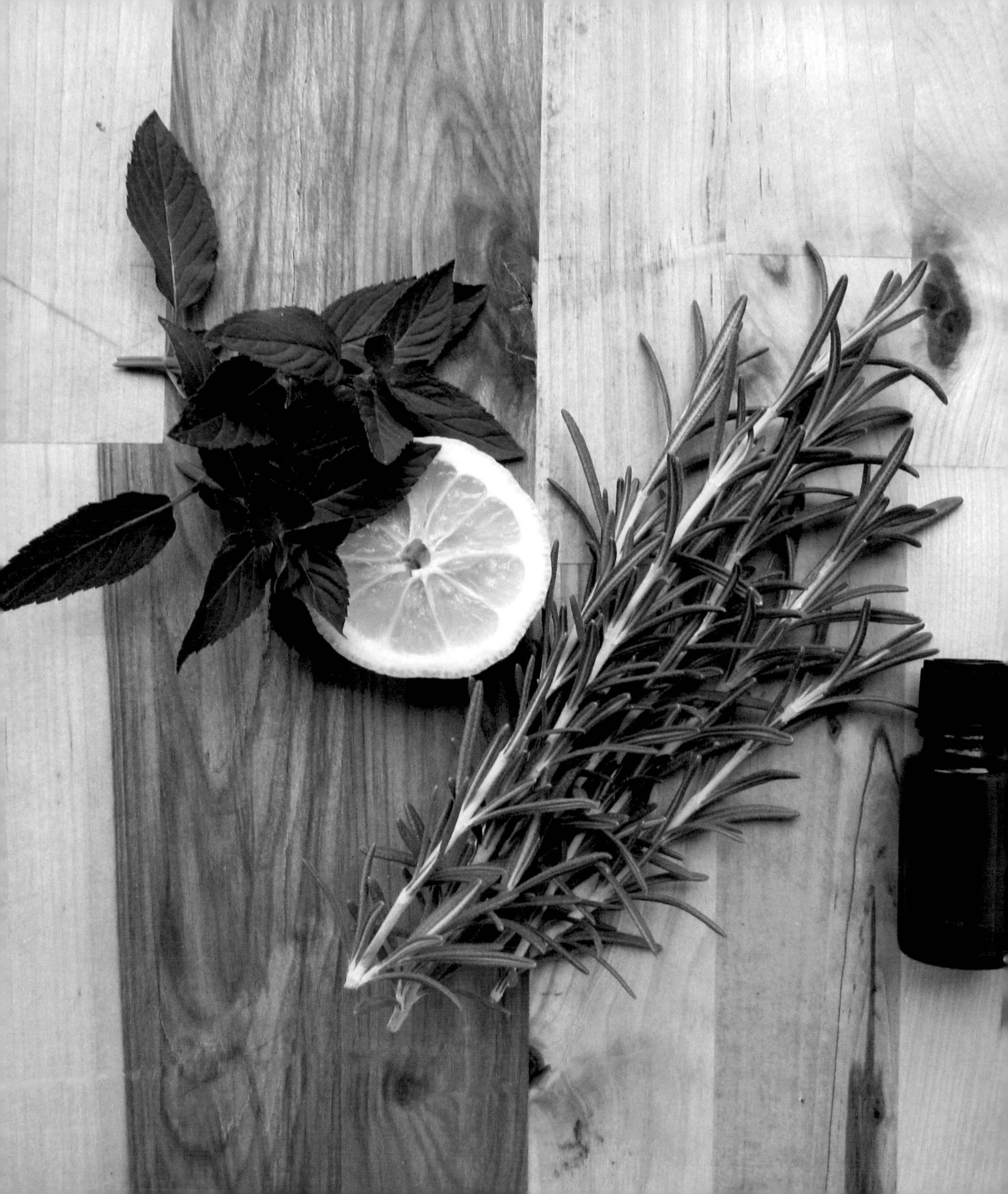

Walk in the Park

- 2 drops Bergamot essential oil
- 2 drops Lemon essential oil
- 1 drop Rosemary essential oil
- 1 drop Peppermint essential oil

"Gee, Your House Smells Terrific"

- 2 drops Lemon essential oil
- 1 drop Cilantro essential oil
- 1 drop Lime essential oil
- 1 drop Melaleuca essential oil

11

Relaxation & Sleep

Great sleep begins before your head hits the pillow. These diffuser combos promote relaxation and decrease stress—things we can all benefit from.

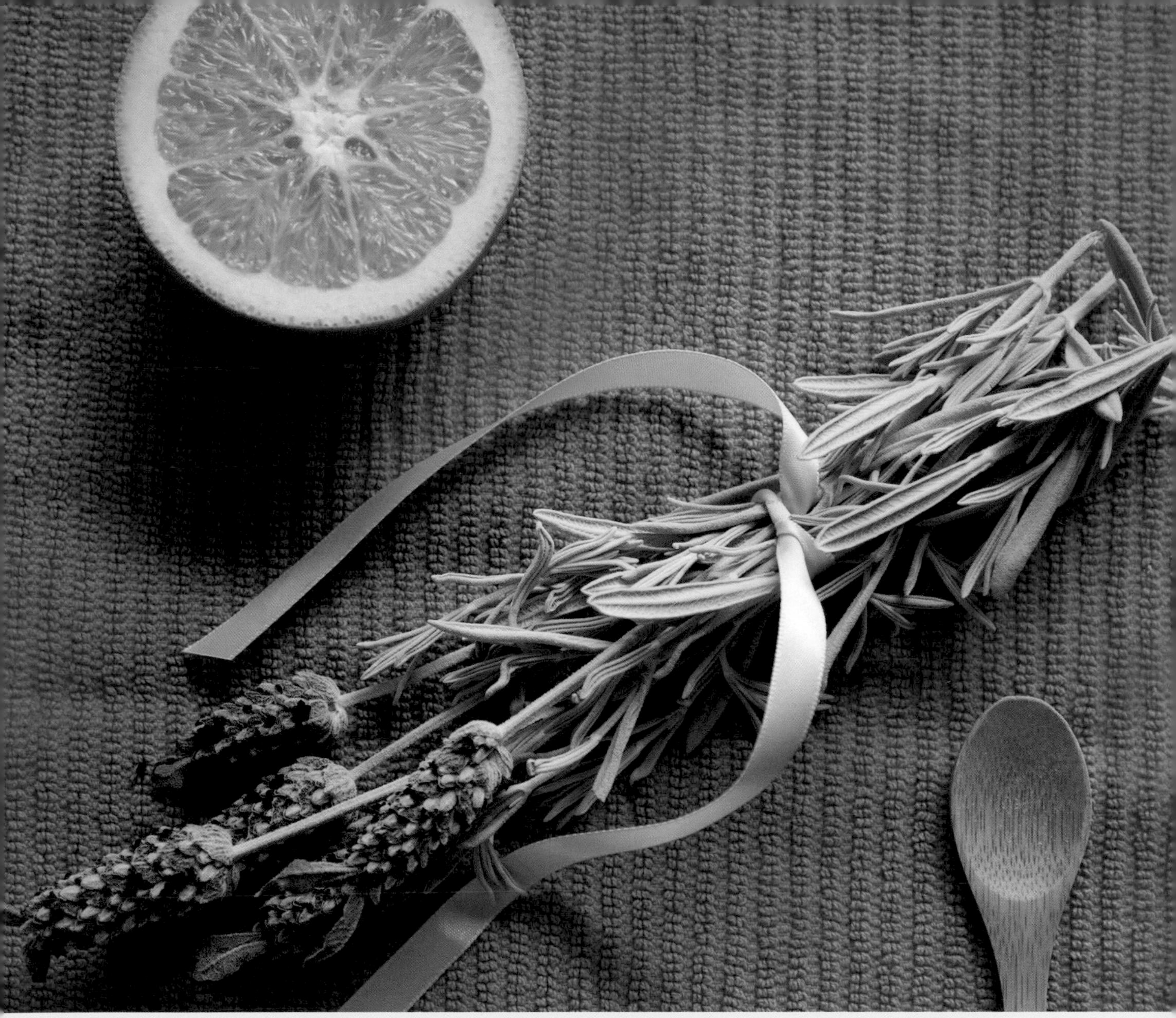

Lavender Lullaby

- 2 drops Lavender essential oil
- 2 drops Vetiver essential oil
- 2 drops Wild Orange essential oil

Peaceful Forest

- 4 drops Lavender essential oil
- 2 drops Cedarwood essential oil

Sleepy Baby

- 2 drops Lavender essential oil
- 1 drop Roman Chamomile essential oil
- 1 drop Vetiver essential oil

Fireflies

- 3 drops Sandalwood essential oil
- 2 drops Ylang Ylang essential oil

Dreamweaver

- 3 drops Cedarwood essential oil
- 3 drops Patchouli essential oil

Blue Moon

- 3 drops Blue Tansy essential oil
- 2 drops Cedarwood essential oil
- 1 drop Lavender essential oil

Be Still

- 3 drops Frankincense essential oil
- 2 drops Vetiver essential oil

Rest for Mama

- 3 drops Roman Chamomile essential oil
- 1 drop Clary Sage essential oil
- 1 drop Bergamot essential oil

Quiet Mind

- 3 drops Bergamot essential oil
- 2 drops Cedarwood essential oil
- 2 drops Sandalwood essential oil

Delightful Calm

- 3 drops Patchouli essential oil
- 2 drops Frankincense essential oil
- 2 drops Wild Orange essential oil

Destination Moon

- 2 drops Lavender essential oil
- 2 drops Wild Orange essential oil
- 1 drop Clary Sage essential oil
- 1 drop Geranium essential oil

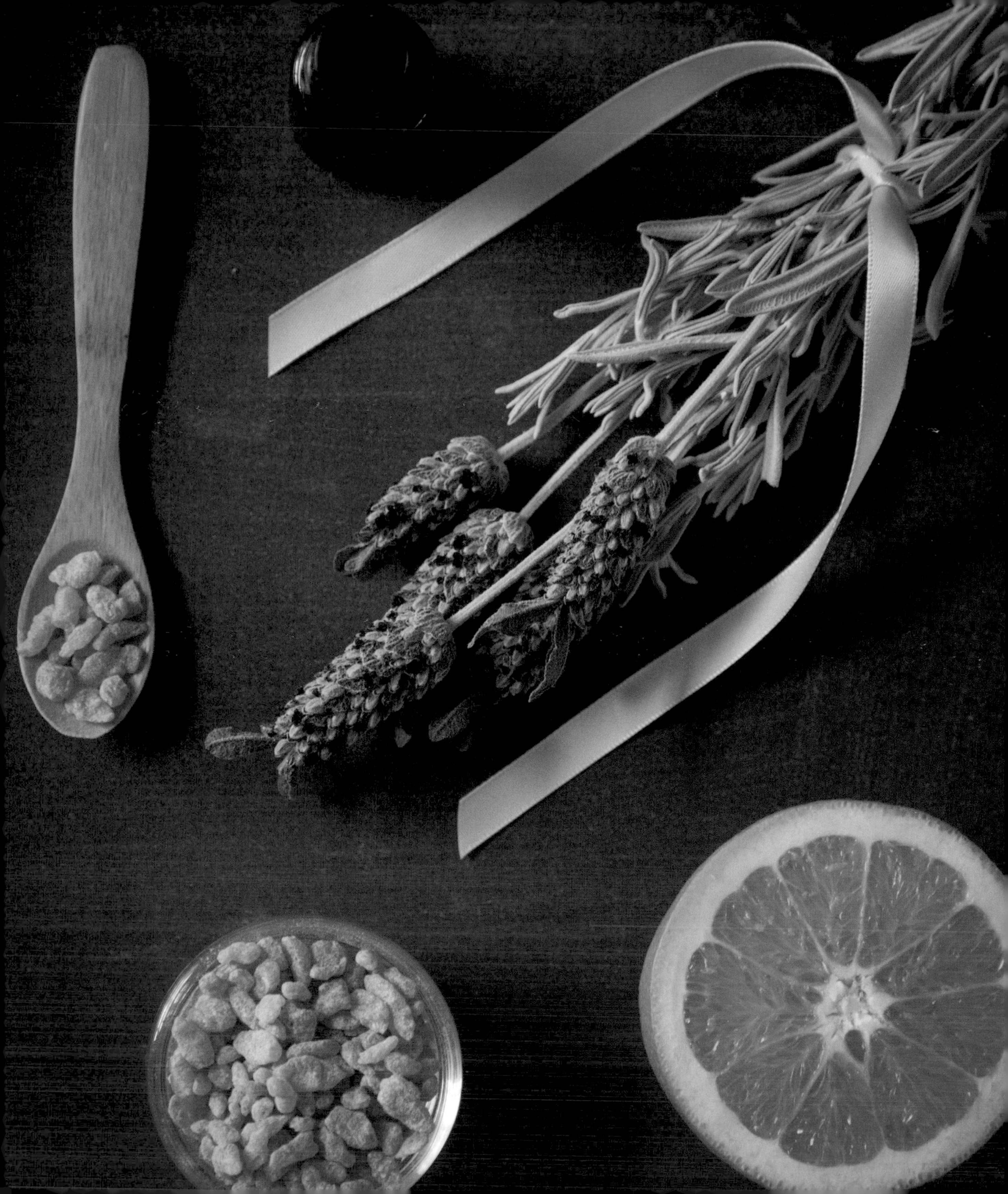

Perfectly Peaceful

- 2 drops Lavender essential oil
- 2 drops Marjoram essential oil
- 2 drops Wild Orange essential oil
- 1 drop Roman Chamomile essential oil

Sweet Slumber

- 2 drops Lavender essential oil
- 2 drops Sandalwood essential oil
- 2 drops Vetiver essential oil
- 1 drop Ylang Ylang essential oil

Hibernate

- 2 drops Lavender essential oil
- 2 drops Wild Orange essential oil
- 1 drop Clary Sage essential oil
- 1 drop Frankincense essential oil

12

Seasonal Support

These recipes come in handy to support healthy respiratory function in the spring and summer, and to keep pesky insects away when you're camping, hiking, or having a picnic.

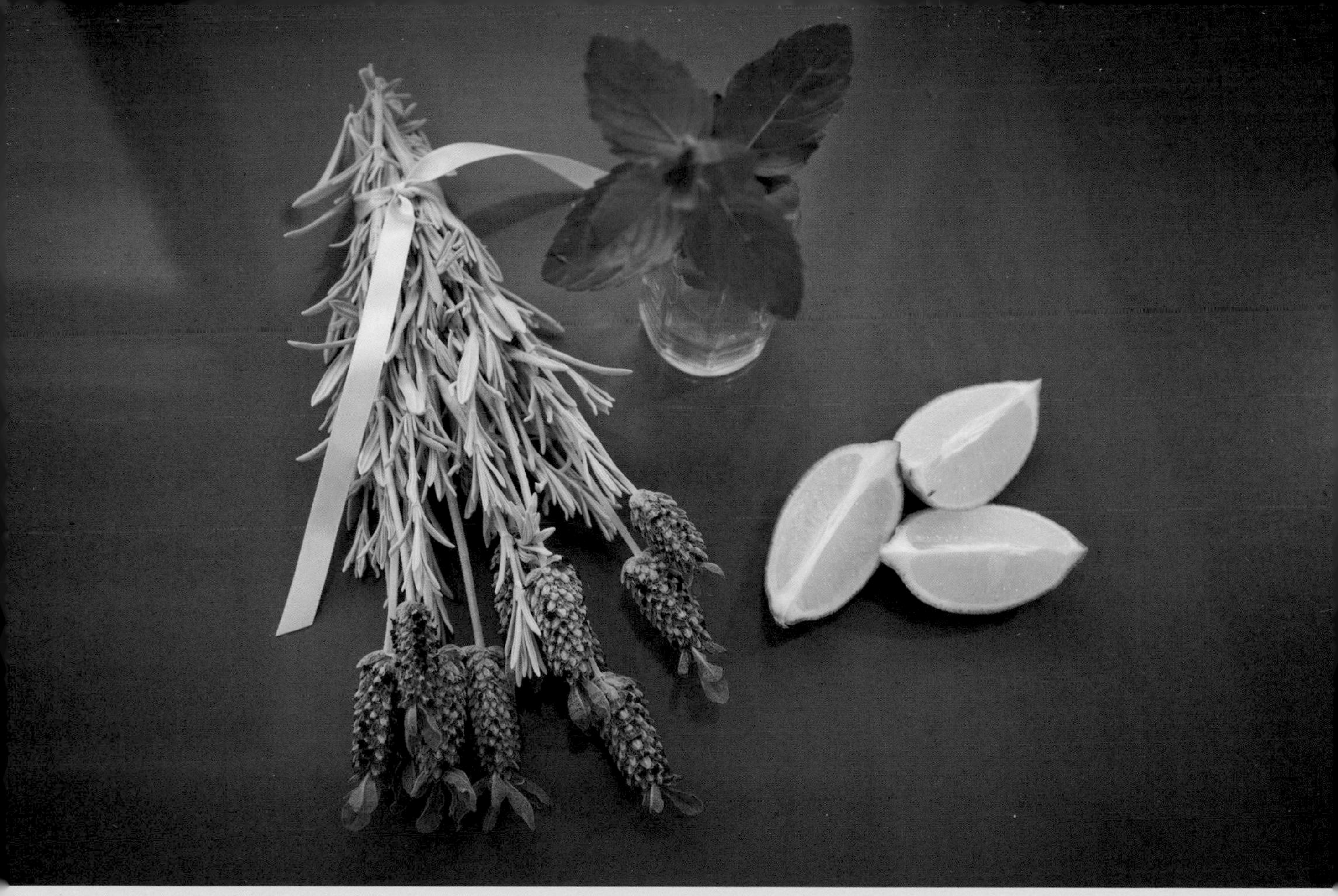

No More Sniffles

- 2 drops Lavender essential oil
- 2 drops Lemon essential oil
- 2 drops Melaleuca essential oil
- 2 drops Peppermint essential oil

Breathe Freely

- 2 drops Peppermint essential oil
- 1 drop Eucalyptus essential oil
- 1 drop Lemon essential oil
- 1 drop Rosemary essential oil

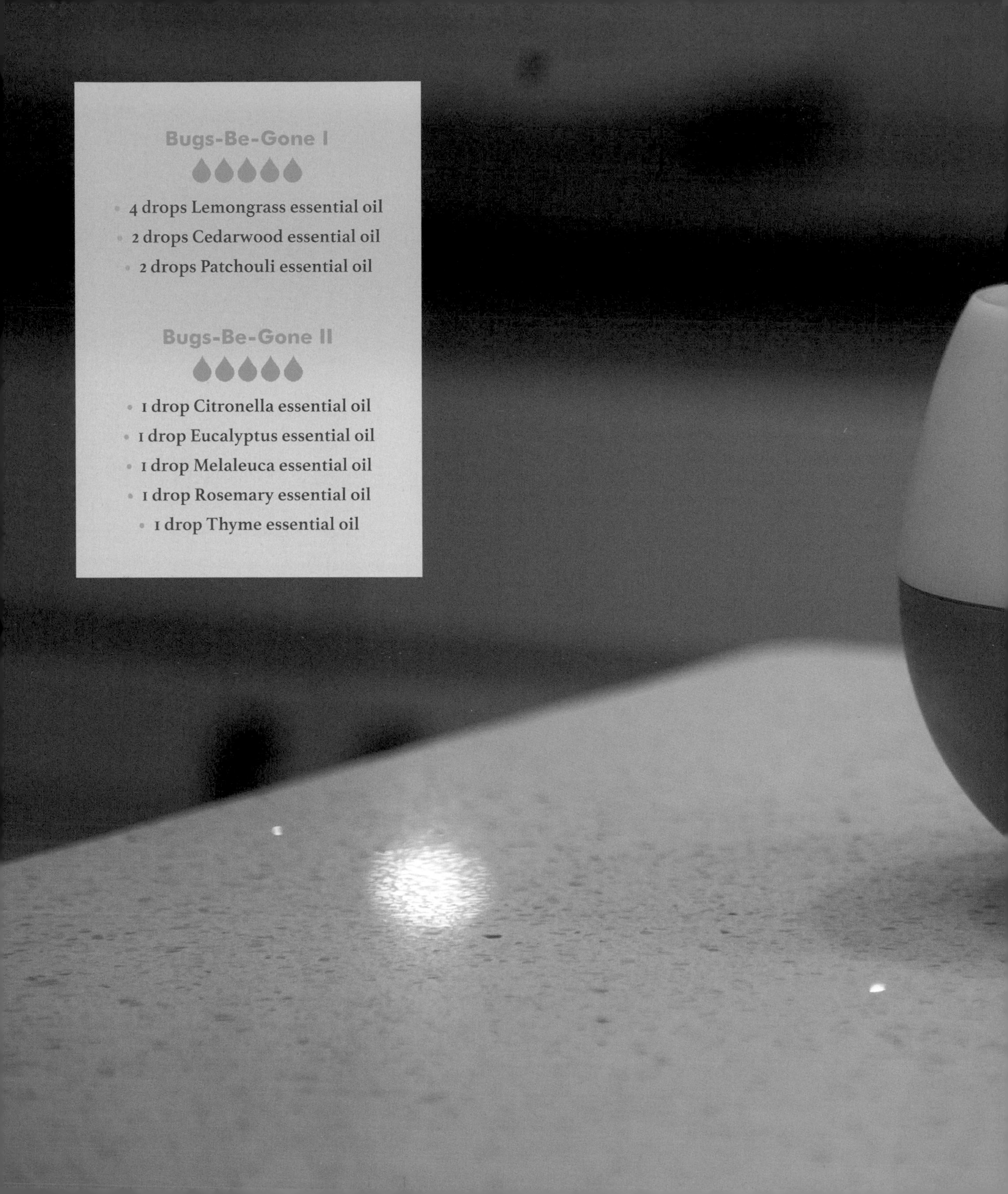

Bugs-Be-Gone I

- 4 drops Lemongrass essential oil
- 2 drops Cedarwood essential oil
- 2 drops Patchouli essential oil

Bugs-Be-Gone II

- 1 drop Citronella essential oil
- 1 drop Eucalyptus essential oil
- 1 drop Melaleuca essential oil
- 1 drop Rosemary essential oil
- 1 drop Thyme essential oil

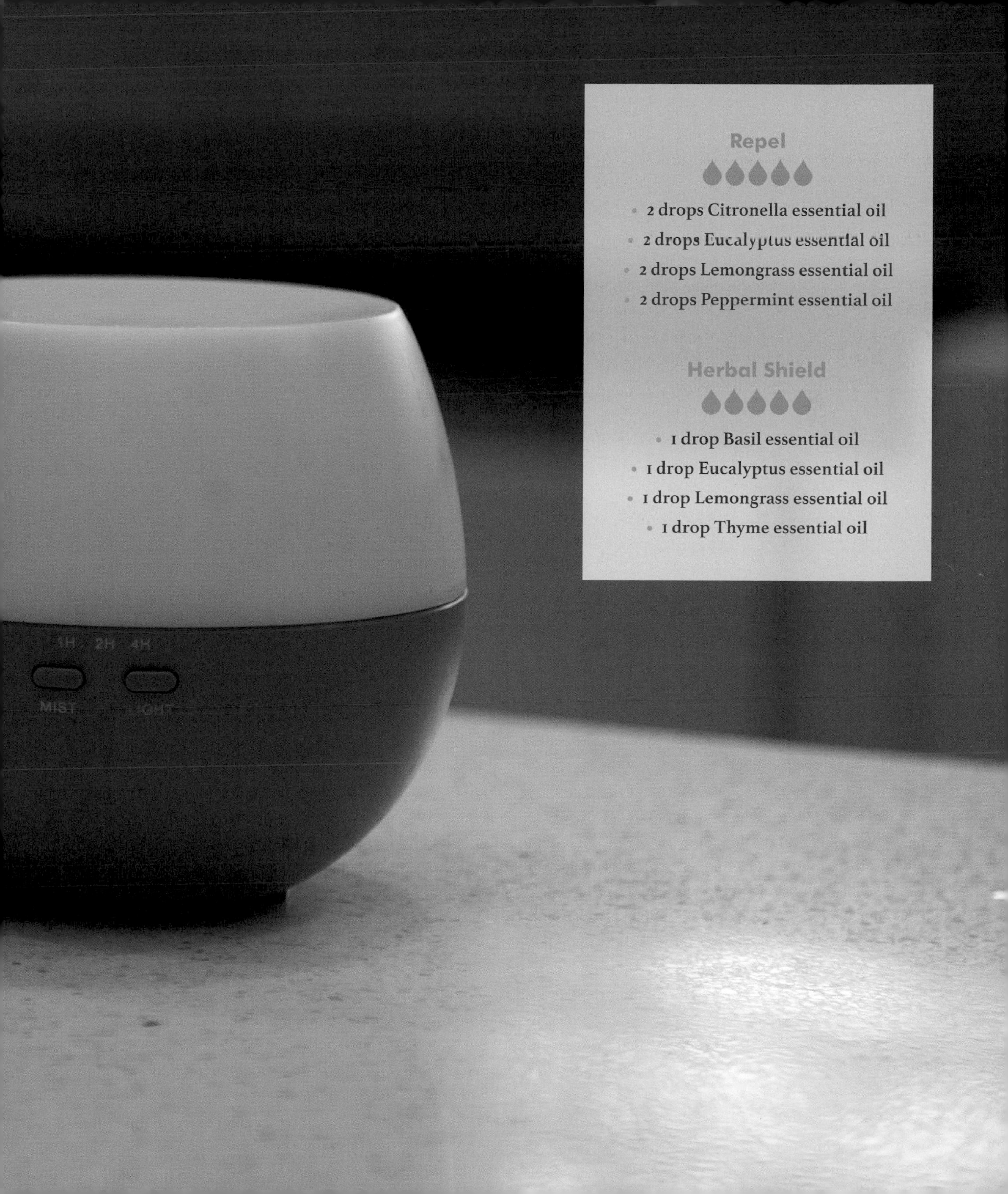

Repel

- 2 drops Citronella essential oil
- 2 drops Eucalyptus essential oil
- 2 drops Lemongrass essential oil
- 2 drops Peppermint essential oil

Herbal Shield

- 1 drop Basil essential oil
- 1 drop Eucalyptus essential oil
- 1 drop Lemongrass essential oil
- 1 drop Thyme essential oil

13

Immune Support

These blends are great to diffuse at the office, the kids' school/daycare, or at home during the fall and winter for immune support.

Wellness Boost I

- 2 drops Douglas Fir essential oil
- 2 drops Eucalyptus essential oil
- 1 drop Peppermint essential oil

Wellness Boost II

- 3 drops Arborvitae essential oil
- 2 drops Cardamom essential oil
- 2 drops Cassia essential oil

Respiratory Relief

- 2 drops Cardamom essential oil
- 2 drops Tangerine essential oil
- 1 drop Dill essential oil

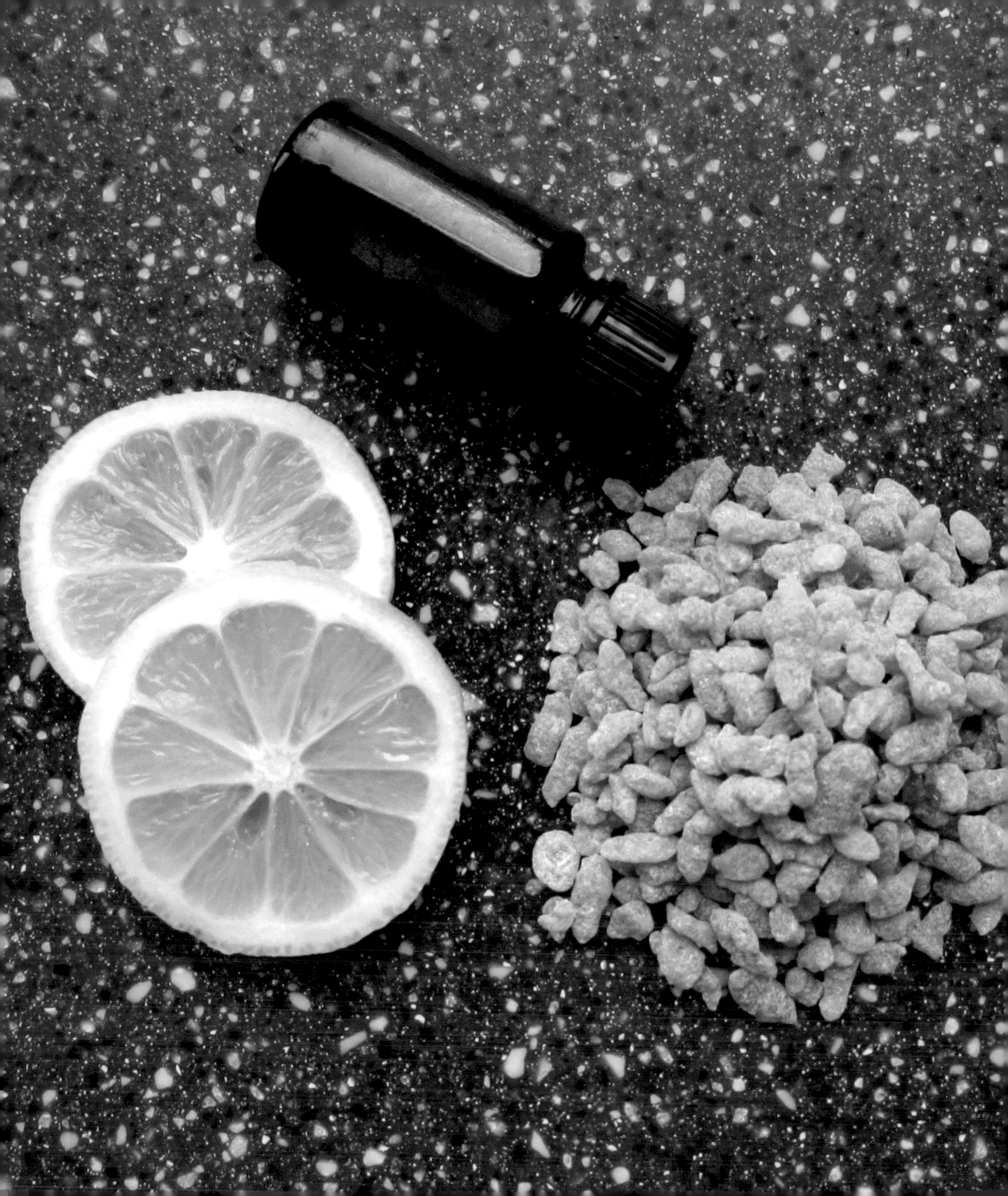

Shields Up

- 4 drops Lemon essential oil
- 3 drops Frankincense essential oil
- 1 drop Arborvitae essential oil

Healthy Body

- 1 drop Eucalyptus essential oil
- 1 drop Lemon essential oil
- 1 drop Lime essential oil
- 1 drop Peppermint essential oil
- 1 drop Rosemary essential oil

Superhero Health I

- 1 drop Cinnamon Bark essential oil
- 1 drop Clove essential oil
- 1 drop Eucalyptus essential oil
- 1 drop Rosemary essential oil
- 1 drop Wild Orange essential oil

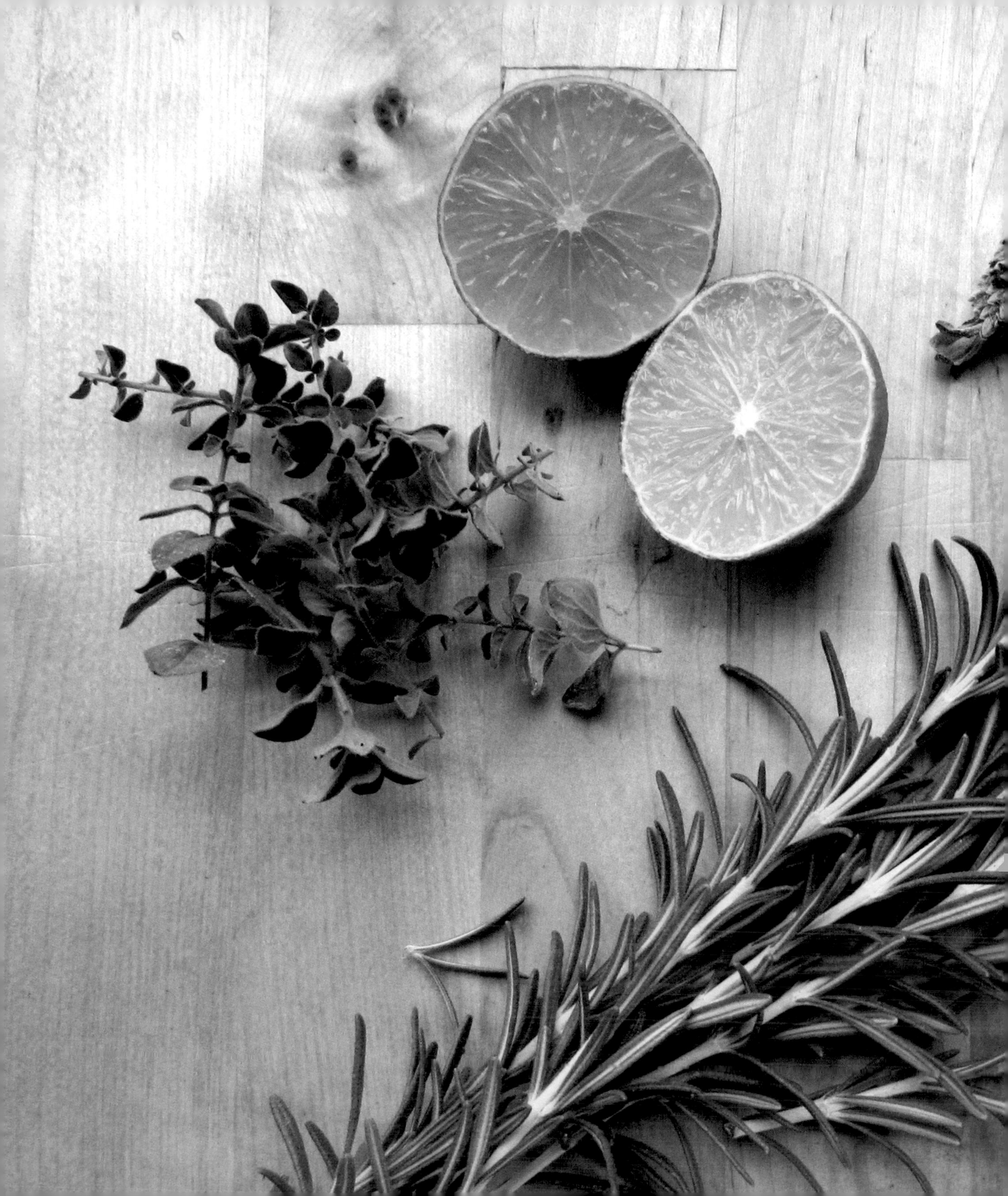

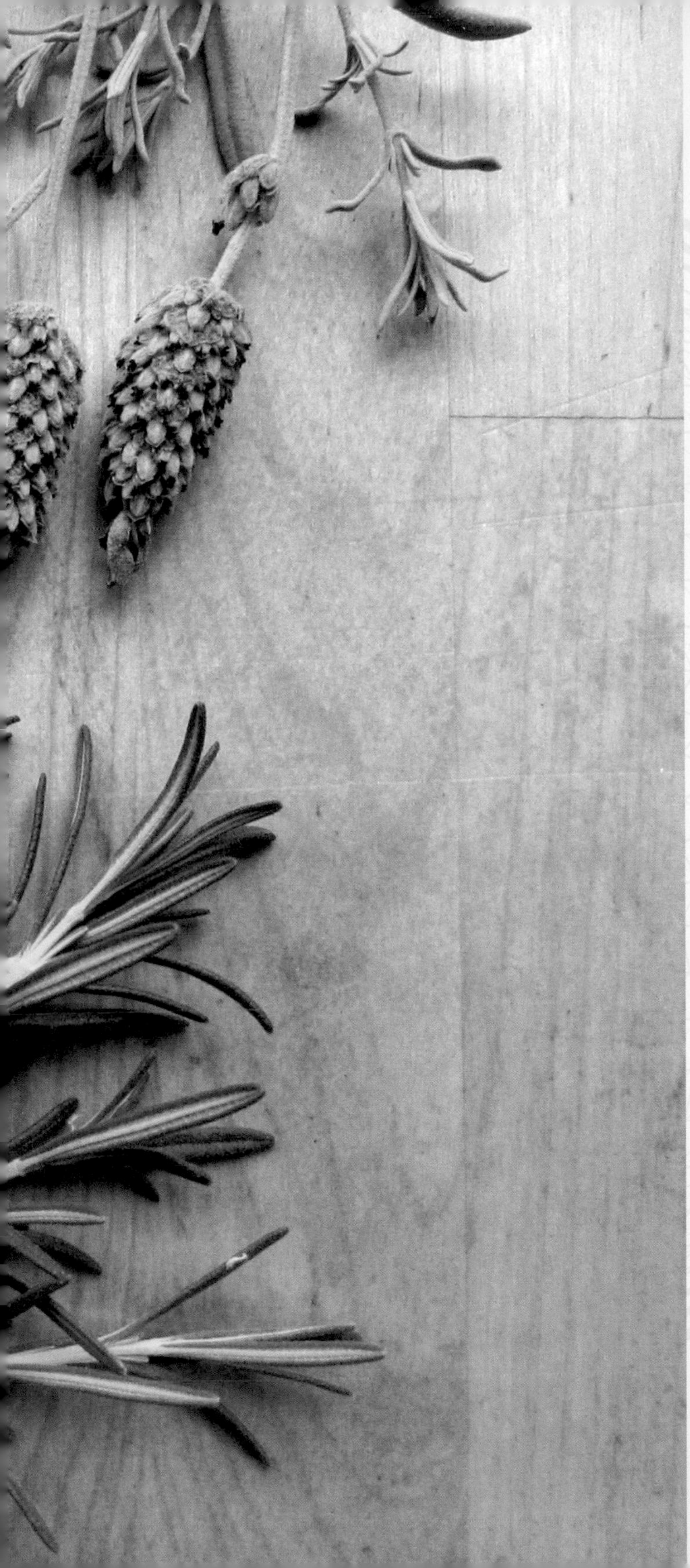

Champion

- 2 drops Lavender essential oil
- 2 drops Lime essential oil
- 1 drop Oregano essential oil
- 1 drop Rosemary essential oil

Superhero Health II

- 1 drop Cardamom essential oil
- 1 drop Eucalyptus essential oil
- 1 drop Lemon essential oil
- 1 drop Melaleuca essential oil
- 1 drop Peppermint essential oil
- 1 drop Rosemary essential oil

Breathe Easy

- 4 drops Eucalyptus essential oil
- 2 drops Ravensara essential oil
- 1 drop Lemon essential oil
- 1 drop Peppermint essential oil
- 1 drop Oregano essential oil

Germ Fighter

- 4 drops Clove essential oil
- 3 drops Wild Orange essential oil
- 2 drops Cinnamon Bark essential oil
- 2 drops Eucalyptus essential oil
- 1 drop Rosemary essential oil

14

Just for the Guys

Sometimes men think that essential oils are just for ladies. Essential oils are great for everyone, and the guys in your life will love these diffuser combos.

Man Cave

- 2 drops Cypress essential oil
- 2 drops White Fir essential oil
- 2 drops Wintergreen essential oil

Strong Silent Type

- 2 drops Grapefruit essential oil
- 2 drops Juniper Berry essential oil
- 1 drop Douglas Fir essential oil

Into the Woods

- 2 drops Frankincense essential oil
- 1 drop Arborvitae essential oil
- 1 drop Cedarwood essential oil

Black Licorice

- 3 drops Bergamot essential oil
- 1 drop Basil essential oil
- 1 drop Fennel essential oil

Take a Hike

- 4 drops Wintergreen essential oil
- 2 drops Lemongrass essential oil
- 2 drops Juniper Berry essential oil

Spiced Cider

- 3 drops Wild Orange essential oil
- 2 drops Cinnamon Bark essential oil
- 2 drops Ginger essential oil

Walk in the Woods

- 3 drops Frankincense essential oil
- 2 drops White Fir essential oil
- 1 drop Cedarwood essential oil

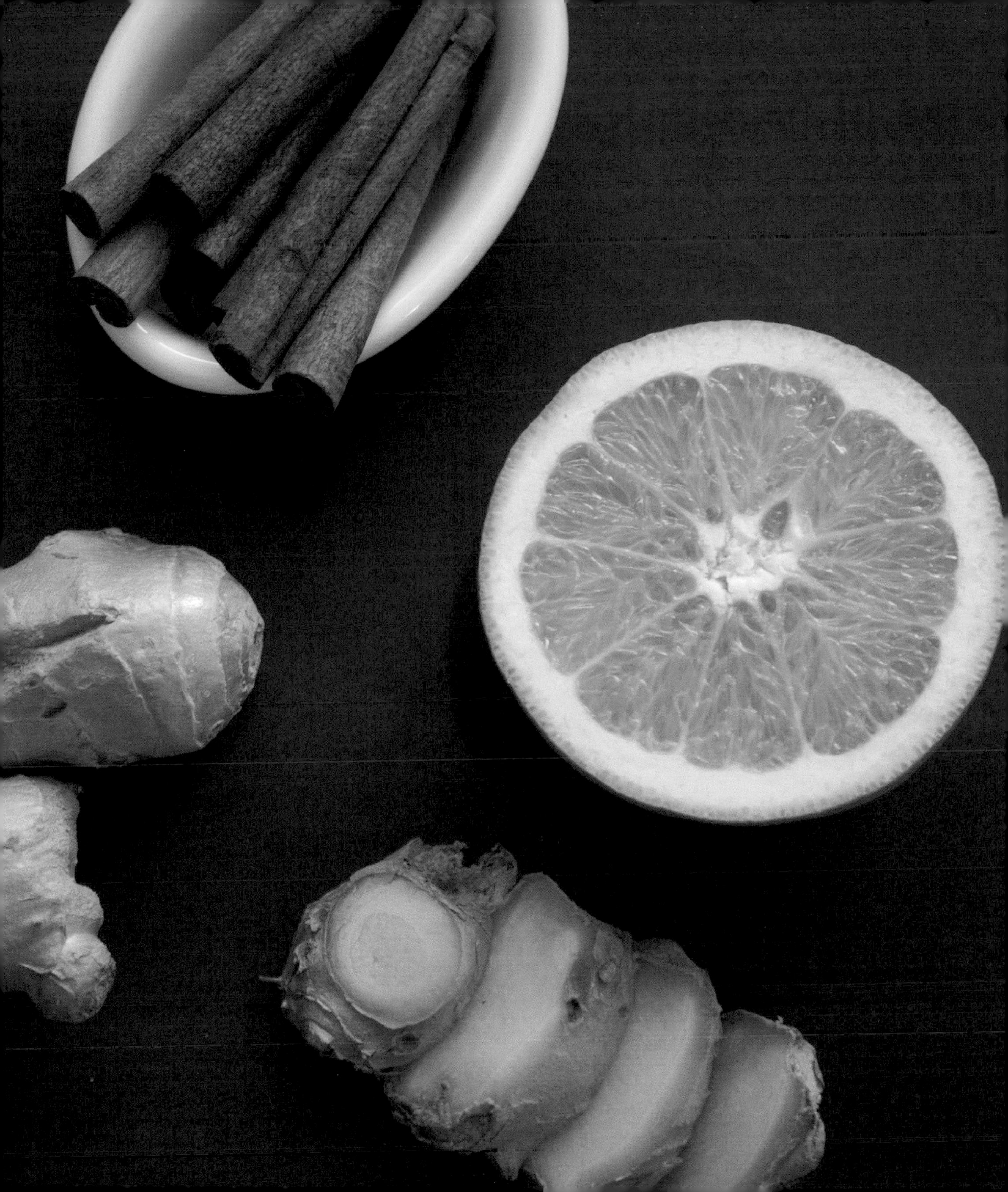

To the Shore

- 2 drops Cedarwood essential oil
- 2 drops Lavender essential oil
- 2 drops Spruce essential oil

The Workshop

- 2 drops Arborvitae essential oil
- 1 drop Douglas Fir essential oil
- 1 drop Spearmint essential oil

Here Comes Your Man

- 3 drops White Fir essential oil
- 2 drops Cardamom essential oil
- 1 drop Arborvitae essential oil
- 1 drop Clove essential oil

Mountain Rain

- 4 drops Cypress essential oil
- 2 drops Cedarwood essential oil
- 2 drops Melaleuca essential oil
- 1 drop Bergamot essential oil

Fire and Ice

- 2 drops Cypress essential oil
- 2 drops Juniper Berry essential oil
- 2 drops White Fir essential oil
- 2 drops Wintergreen essential oil
- 1 drop Cinnamon essential oil

15

Stress Relief

Take control of stress and don't let it control you. Use these diffuser blends when everyone needs to breathe, relax, and chill out.

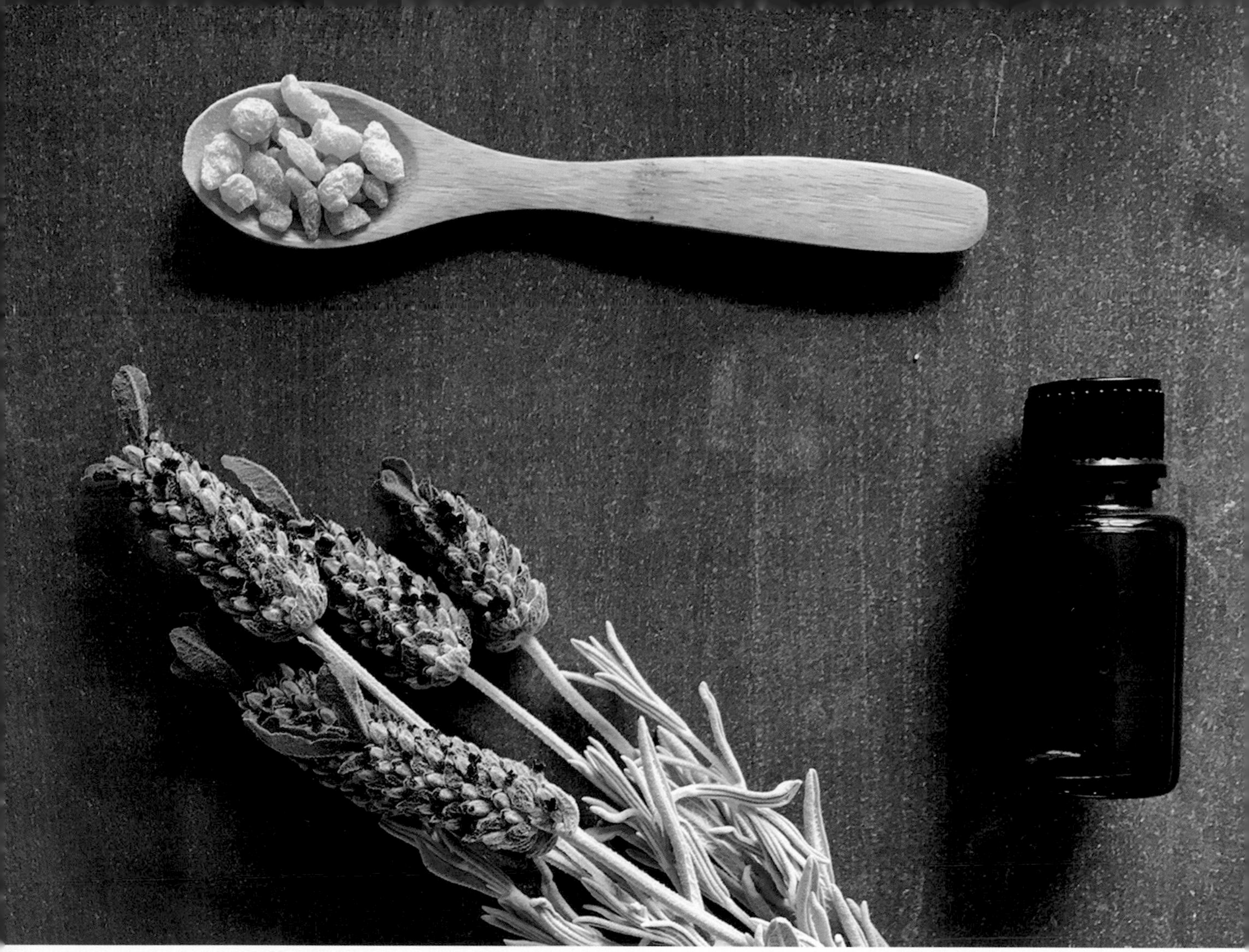

Peace and Calm

- 2 drops Bergamot essential oil
- 2 drops Frankincense essential oil

Quiet Butterfly

- 4 drops Lavender essential oil
- 2 drops Frankincense essential oil

Frayed Nerves

- 2 drops Bergamot essential oil
- 2 drops Patchouli essential oil
- 2 drops Ylang Ylang essential oil

Easy As 1-2-3

- 2 drops Arborvitae essential oil
- 2 drops Bergamot essential oil
- 2 drops Cypress essential oil

Uplifting & Grounding

- 2 drops Eucalyptus essential oil
- 2 drops Lime essential oil
- 2 drops Myrrh essential oil

Stress Less

- 2 drops Bergamot essential oil
- 2 drops Cypress essential oil
- 2 drops Patchouli essential oil

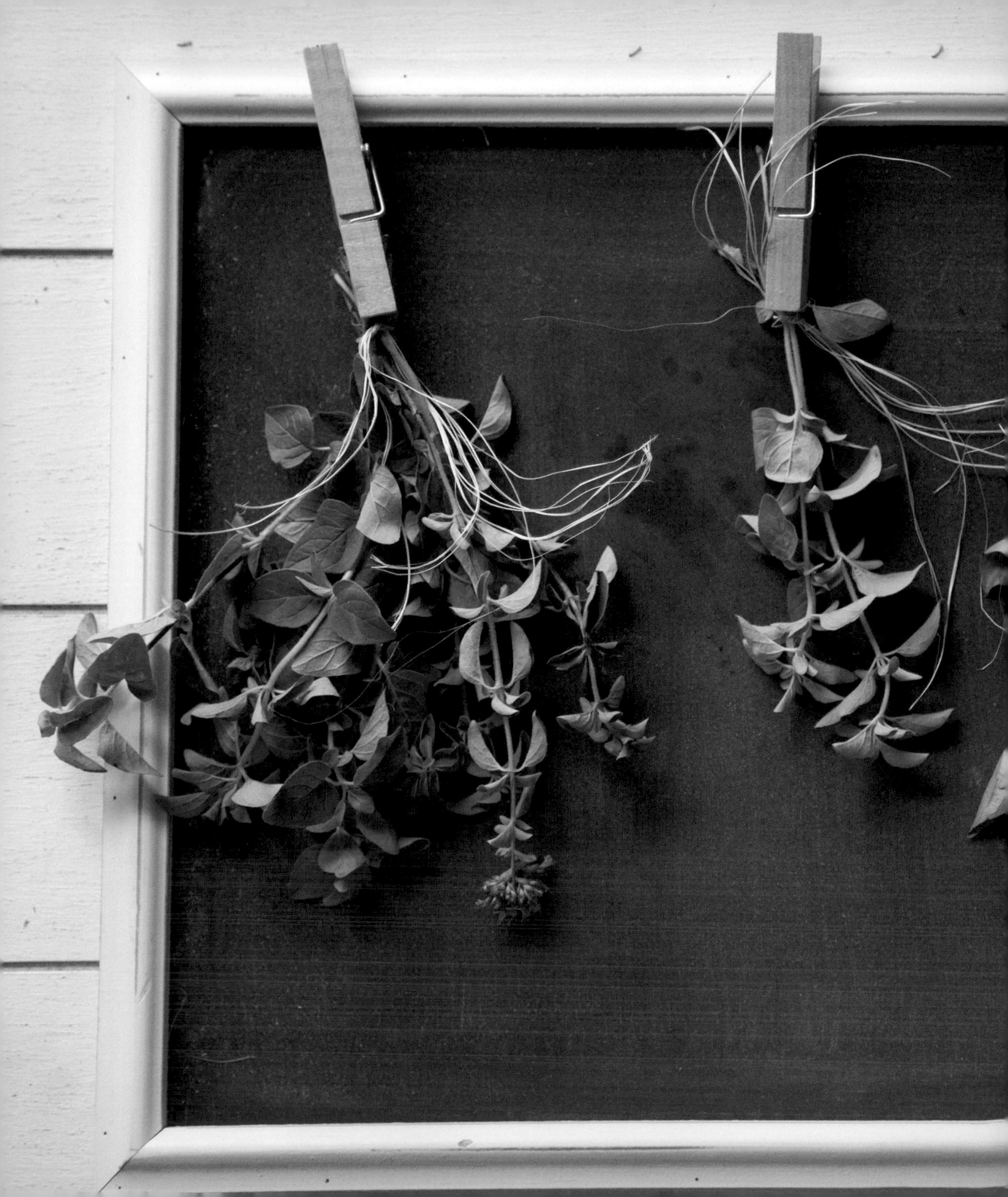

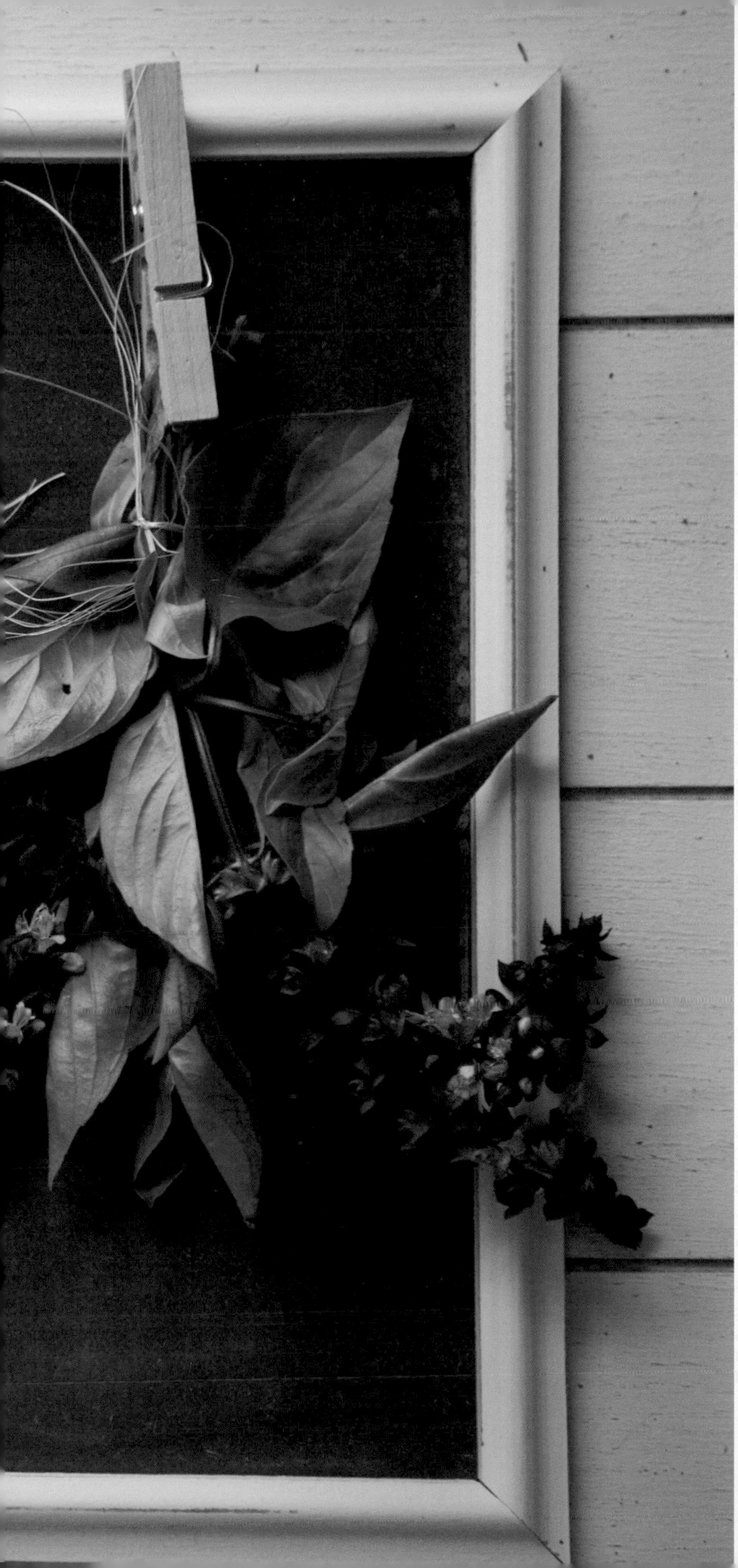

Find Your Zen

- 3 drops Bergamot essential oil
- 1 drop Geranium essential oil
- 1 drop Frankincense essential oil

No More Nerves

- 3 drops Grapefruit essential oil
- 1 drop Jasmine essential oil
- 1 drop Ylang Ylang essential oil

Take it Easy

- 2 drops Myrrh essential oil
- 2 drops Patchouli essential oil
- 2 drops Ylang Ylang essential oil

Gentle Magic

- 3 drops Lavender essential oil
- 2 drops Roman Chamomile essential oil
- 2 drops Ylang Ylang essential oil

Grouch Buster

- 2 drops Cedarwood essential oil
- 2 drops Frankincense essential oil
- 2 drops Wild Orange essential oil
- 1 drop Rosemary essential oil

Be Still

- 3 drops Lavender essential oil
- 1 drop Clary Sage essential oil
- 1 drop Lemon essential oil
- 1 drop Vetiver essential oil

Winding Down

- 4 drops Lavender essential oil
- 2 drops Cedarwood essential oil
- 2 drops Wild Orange essential oil
- 1 drop Ylang Ylang essential oil

Restful Breeze

- 3 drops Clary Sage essential oil
- 3 drops Lavender essential oil
- 2 drops Ylang Ylang essential oil
- 1 drop Marjoram essential oil

16

Romance

Love really IS in the air when you diffuse one of these scintillating combos.

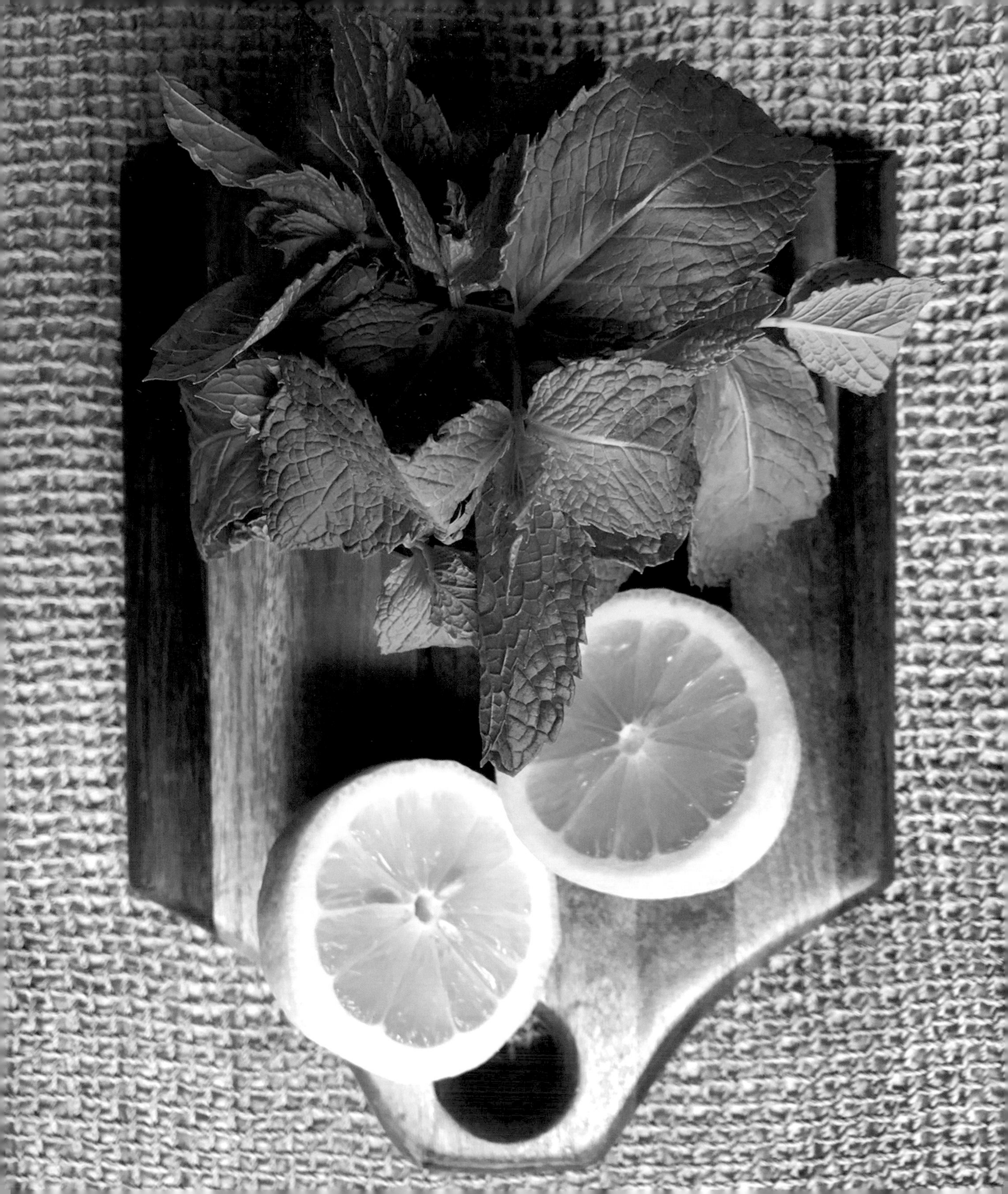

La La Love You

- 4 drops Clary Sage essential oil
- 2 drops Ylang Ylang essential oil

Pillow Talk

- 5 drops Sandalwood essential oil
- 2 drops Vanilla extract
- 1 drop Jasmine essential oil

Angel Shadows

- 3 drops Wintergreen essential oil
- 2 drops Ylang Ylang essential oil
- 1 drop Roman Chamomile essential oil

Be My Valentine

- 2 drops Geranium essential oil
- 2 drops Ylang Ylang essential oil
- 3 drops Lemon essential oil

Light My Fire

- 2 drops Black Pepper essential oil
- 2 drops Grapefruit essential oil
- 2 drops Jasmine essential oil

I'm Yours

- 2 drops Bergamot essential oil
- 2 drops Black Pepper essential oil
- 2 drops Ylang Ylang essential oil

Oooh La La

- 2 drops Ginger essential oil
- 2 drops Patchouli essential oil
- 2 drops Ylang Ylang essential oil

Date Night

- 2 drops Wild Orange essential oil
- 1 drop Vetiver essential oil
- 1 drop Ylang Ylang essential oil

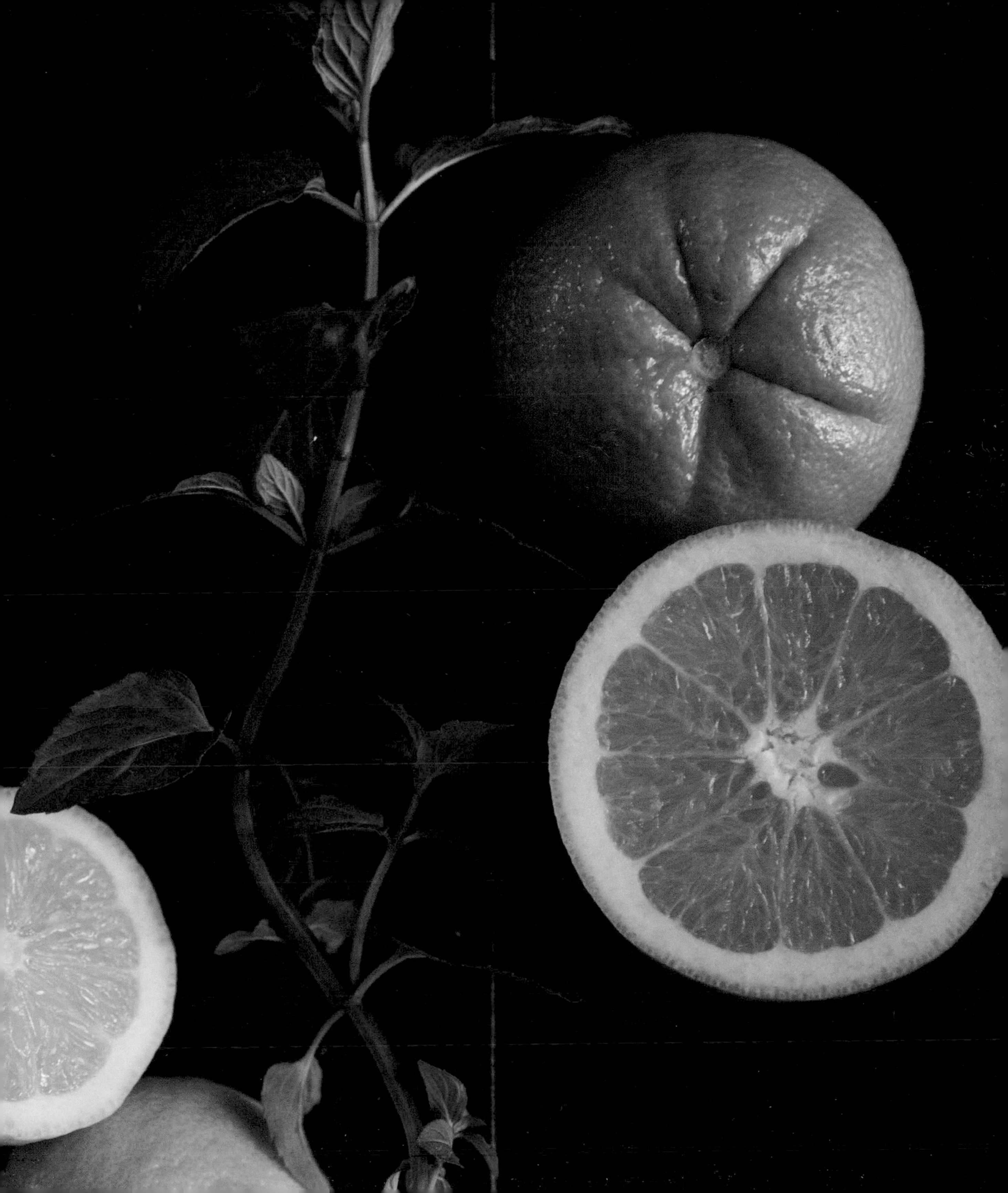

Love Potion

- 4 drops Lavender essential oil
- 1 drop Bergamot essential oil
- 1 drop Patchouli essential oil
- 1 drop Ylang Ylang essential oil

Femme Fatale

- 2 drops Bergamot essential oil
- 2 drops Geranium essential oil
- 2 drops Sandalwood essential oil
- 2 drops Wild Orange essential oil

In the Mood

- 2 drops Coriander essential oil
- 2 drops Sandalwood essential oil
- 2 drops Wild Orange essential oil
- 2 drops Ylang Ylang essential oil

Tranquil Moments

- 2 drops Geranium essential oil
- 2 drops Lavender essential oil
- 1 drop Clary Sage essential oil
- 1 drop Roman Chamomile essential oil
- 1 drop Ylang Ylang essential oil

Come to the Casbah

- 1 drop Cinnamon essential oil
- 1 drop Patchouli essential oil
- 1 drop Rosemary essential oil
- 1 drop Sandalwood essential oil
- 1 drop White Fir essential oil
- 1 drop Ylang Ylang essential oil

17
Spring

Bring the fresh scents of the garden inside with these bright and cheery diffuser blends.

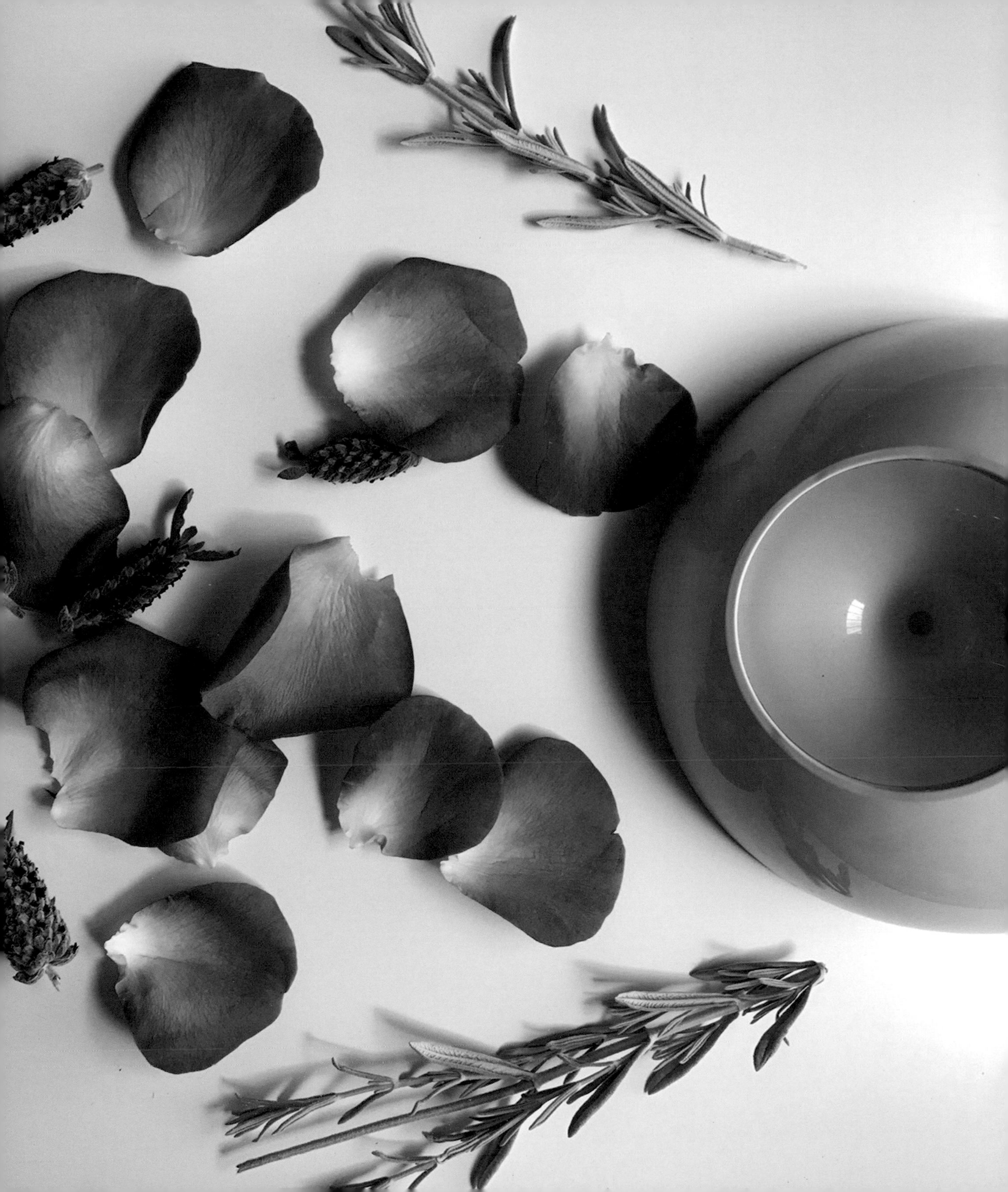

In Full Bloom

- 3 drops Lavender essential oil
- 1 drop Wild Orange essential oil
- 1 drop Rose essential oil

Spring Sunset

- 2 drops Lavender essential oil
- 2 drops Ylang Ylang essential oil
- 1 drop Clary Sage essential oil

Lemon Rain

- 4 drops Lemon essential oil
- 1 drop Vetiver essential oil

Isla de Encanta

- 3 drops Clary Sage essential oil
- 2 drops Cedarwood essential oil
- 2 drops Wild Orange essential oil

Easy Breezy

- 4 drops Grapefruit essential oil
- 2 drops Eucalyptus essential oil
- 2 drops Rosemary essential oil

Freshly Cut Flowers

- 2 drops Basil essential oil
- 2 drops Lavender essential oil
- 2 drops Ylang Ylang essential oil

Spring Rain

- 3 drops Bergamot essential oil
- 2 drops Clary Sage essential oil
- 2 drops Lavender essential oil

Sun-Kissed

- 2 drops Grapefruit essential oil
- 2 drops Juniper Berry essential oil
- 1 drop Wild Orange essential oil

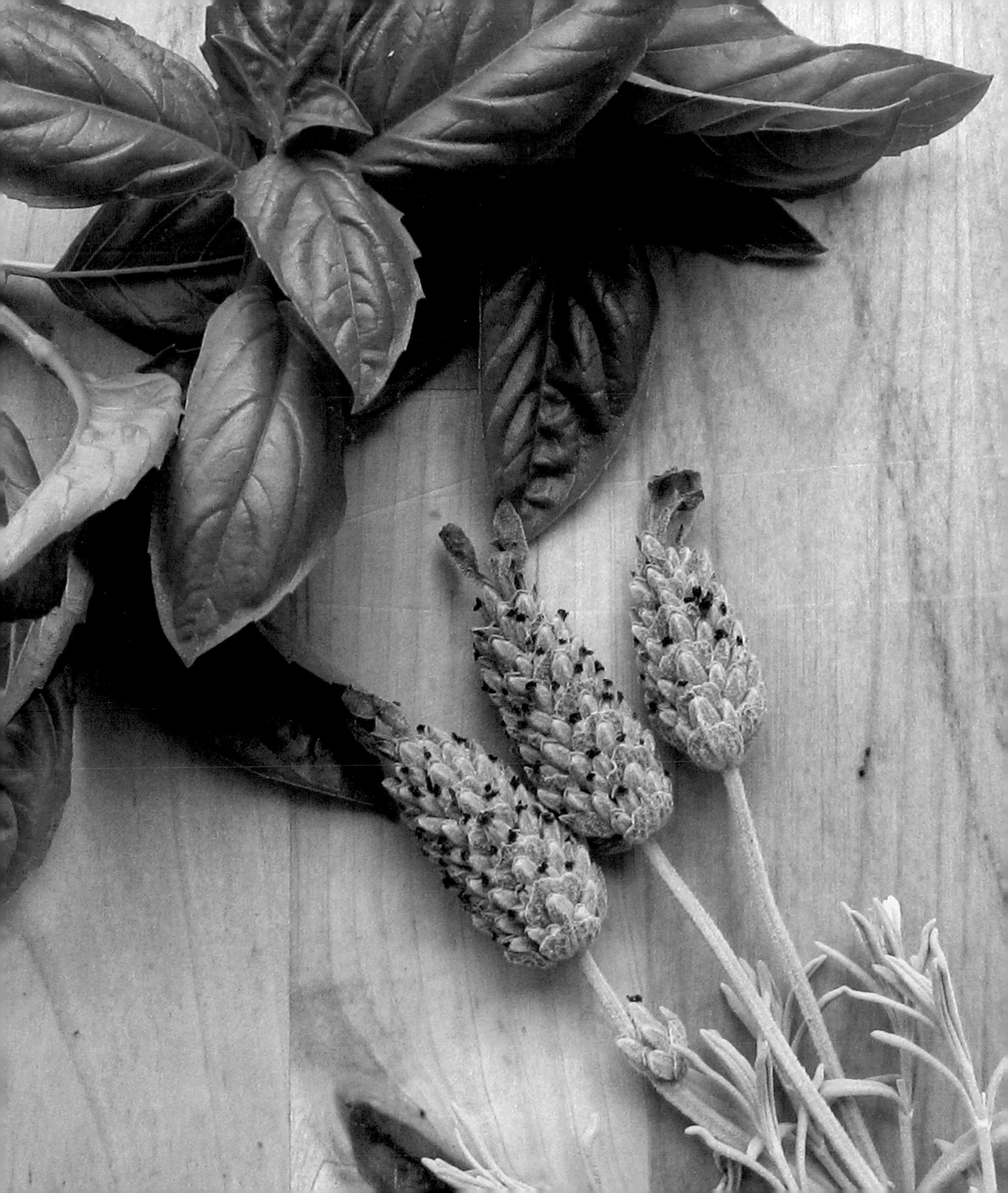

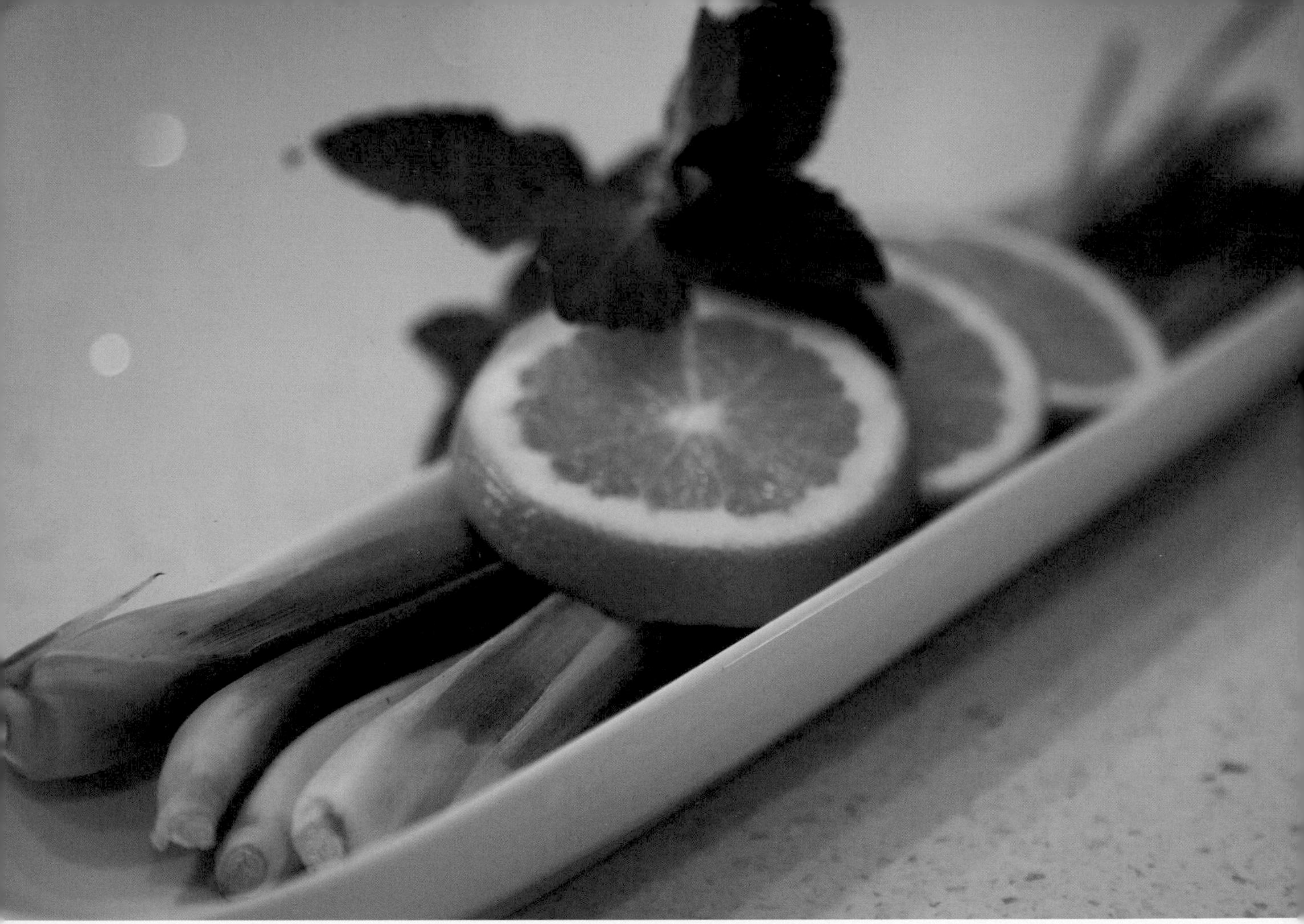

Pixie Dust

- 3 drops Wild Orange essential oil
- 2 drops Spearmint essential oil
- 1 drop Lemongrass essential oil

Citrus Sunrise

- 2 drops Bergamot essential oil
- 2 drops Lemon essential oil
- 2 drops Wild Orange essential oil

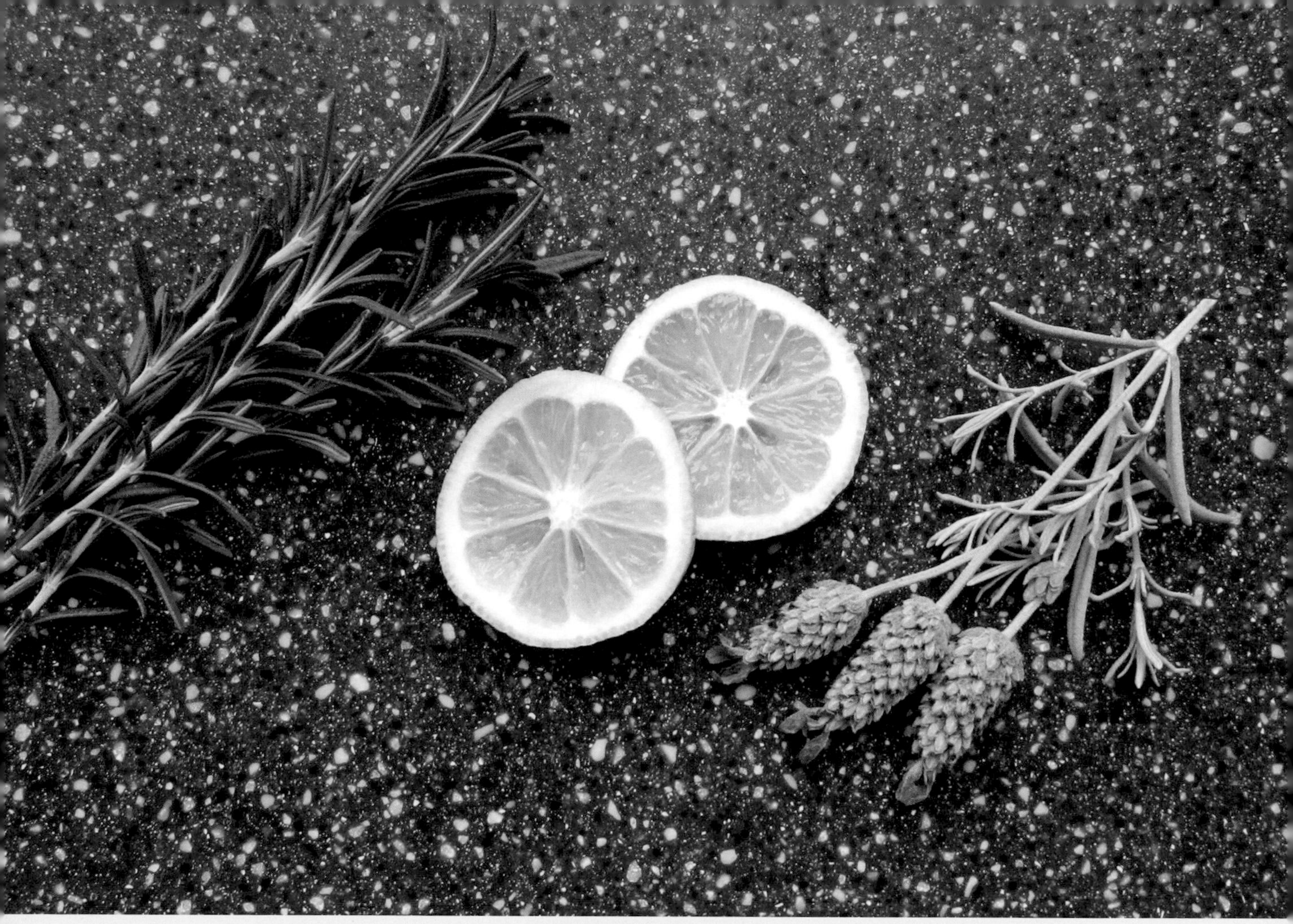

Happy Mom

- 2 drops Arborvitae essential oil
- 2 drops Bergamot essential oil
- 2 drops Wild Orange essential oil

Fresh and Clean

- 2 drops Lavender essential oil
- 2 drops Lemon essential oil
- 2 drops Rosemary essential oil

End of the Rainbow

- 1 drop Bergamot essential oil
- 1 drop Lavender essential oil
- 1 drop Rosemary essential oil
- 1 drop Peppermint essential oil
- 1 drop Wild Orange essential oil
- 1 drop Ylang Ylang essential oil

18

Summer

These diffuser combos will transport you to a warm, sandy beach with a cool drink in your hand.

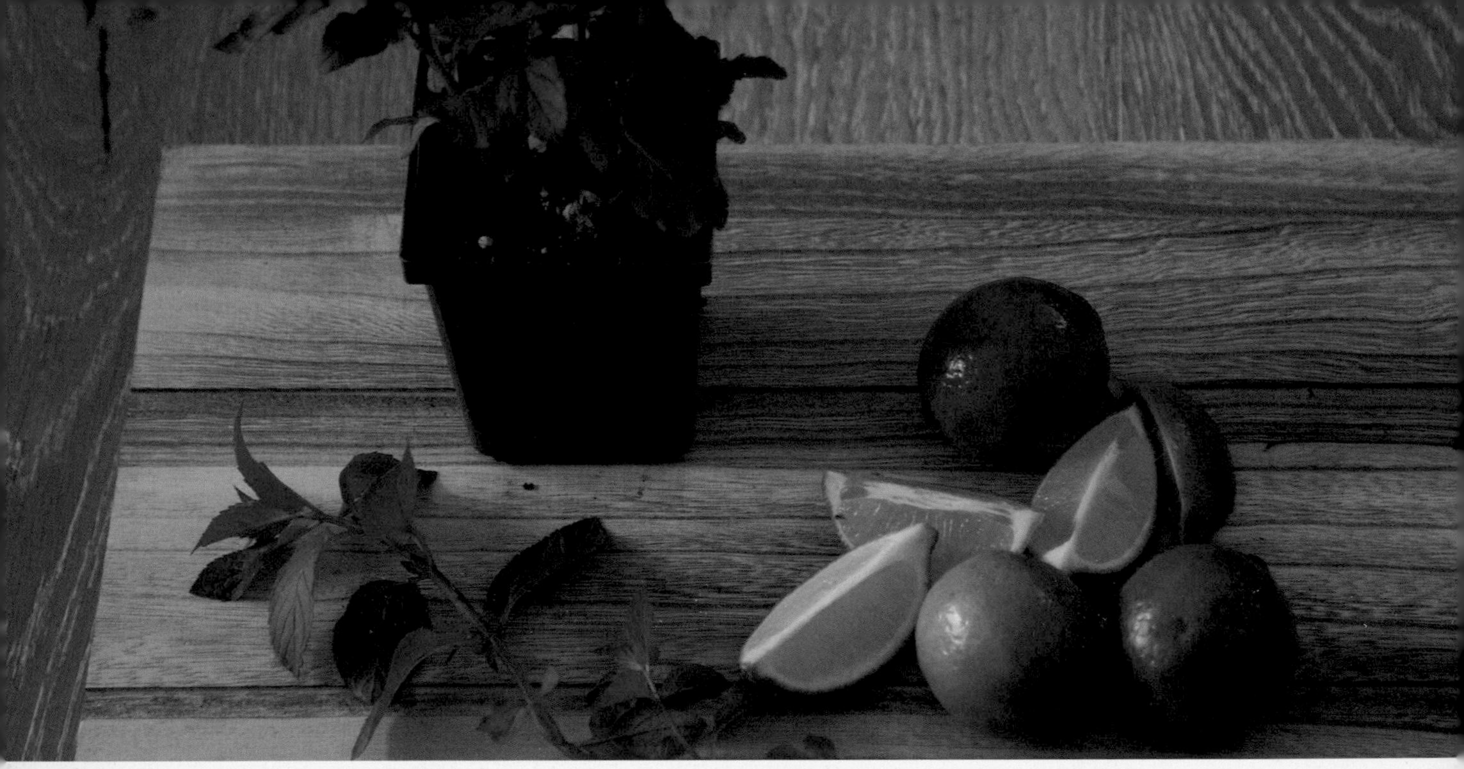

Fresh Mojito

- 2 drops Lime essential oil
- 2 drops Peppermint essential oil
- 1 drop Spearmint essential oil

Rocky Mountain High

- 2 drops Lemon essential oil
- 2 drops Peppermint essential oil
- 1 drop Ylang Ylang essential oil

Coastal Waters

- 3 drops Lavender essential oil
- 3 drops Lime essential oil
- 1 drop Spearmint essential oil

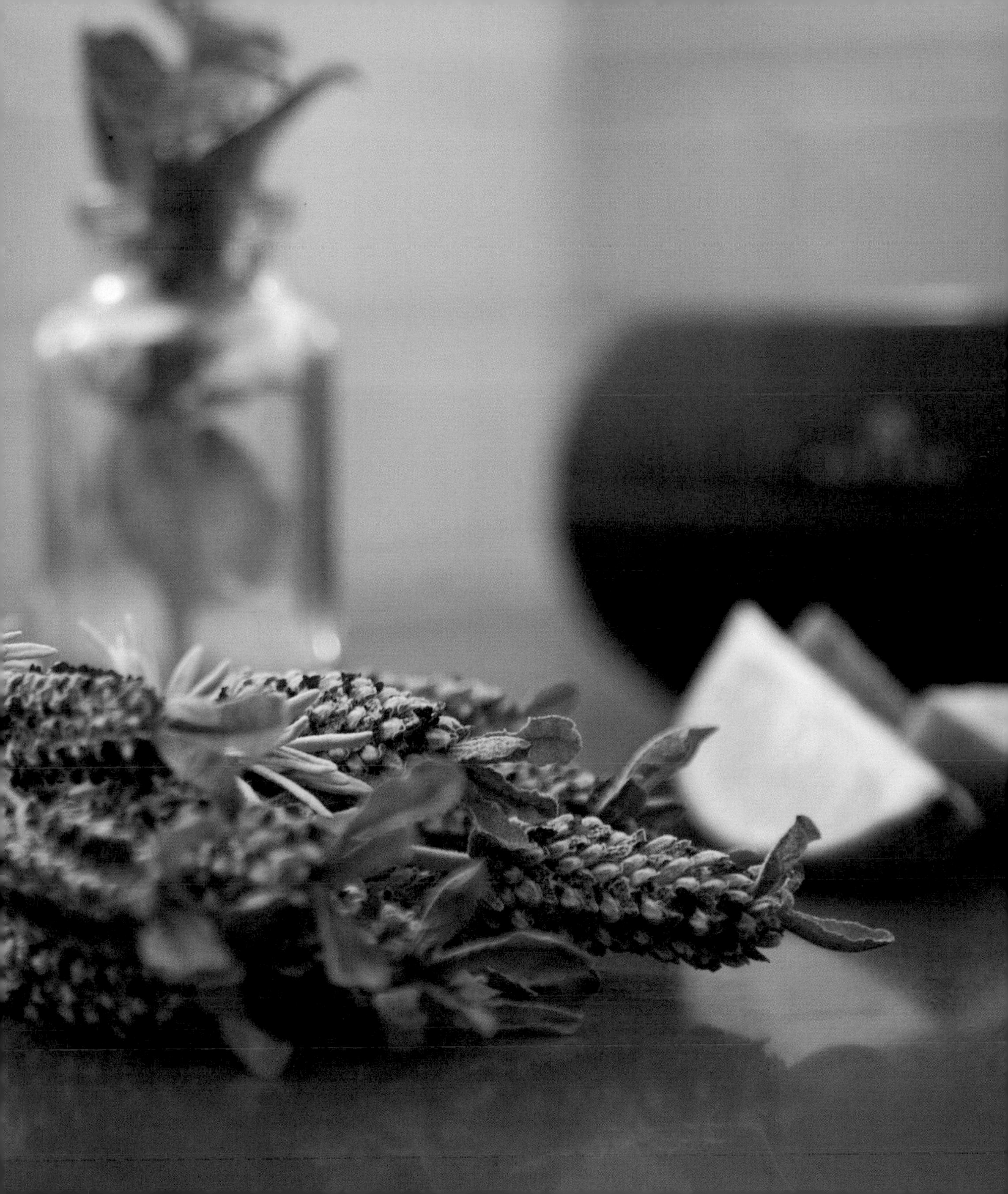

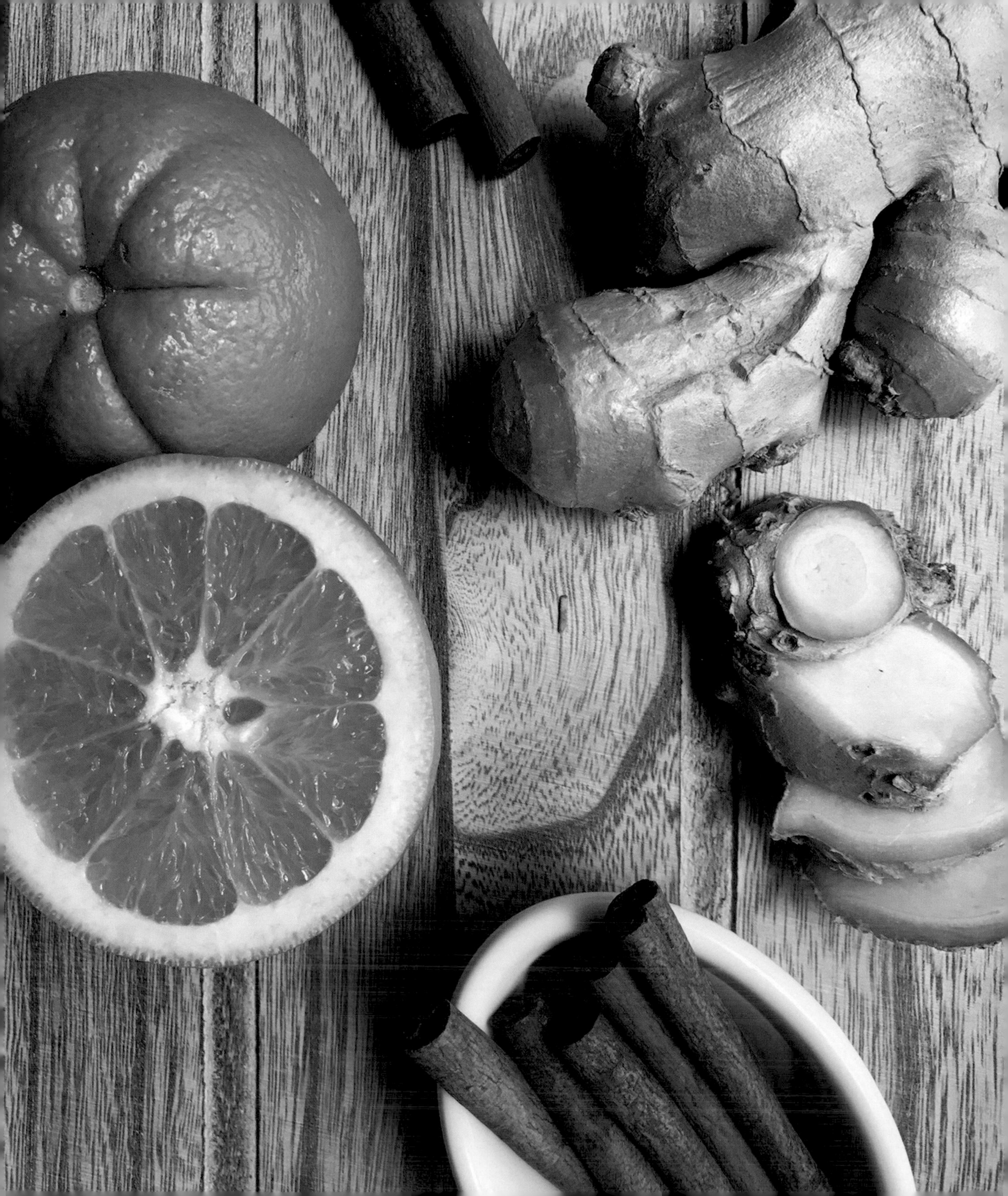

Summer Lovin'

- 3 drops Wild Orange essential oil
- 2 drops Bergamot essential oil
- 2 drops Ylang Ylang essential oil

Let the Sun Shine In

- 3 drops Wild Orange essential oil
- 2 drops Bergamot essential oil
- 1 drop Patchouli essential oil

Picnic Time

- 3 drops Spearmint essential oil
- 2 drops Dill essential oil
- 1 drop Lemongrass essential oil

Hawaiian Sun

- 3 drops Wild Orange essential oil
- 2 drops Ginger essential oil
- 2 drops Ylang Ylang essential oil

Just Like Paradise

- 3 drops Grapefruit essential oil
- 2 drops Sandalwood essential oil
- 2 drops Wild Orange essential oil
- 1 drop vanilla extract

Sea Breezes

- 2 drops Bergamot essential oil
- 2 drops Lavender essential oil
- 1 drop Rosemary essential oil
- 1 drop Eucalyptus essential oil

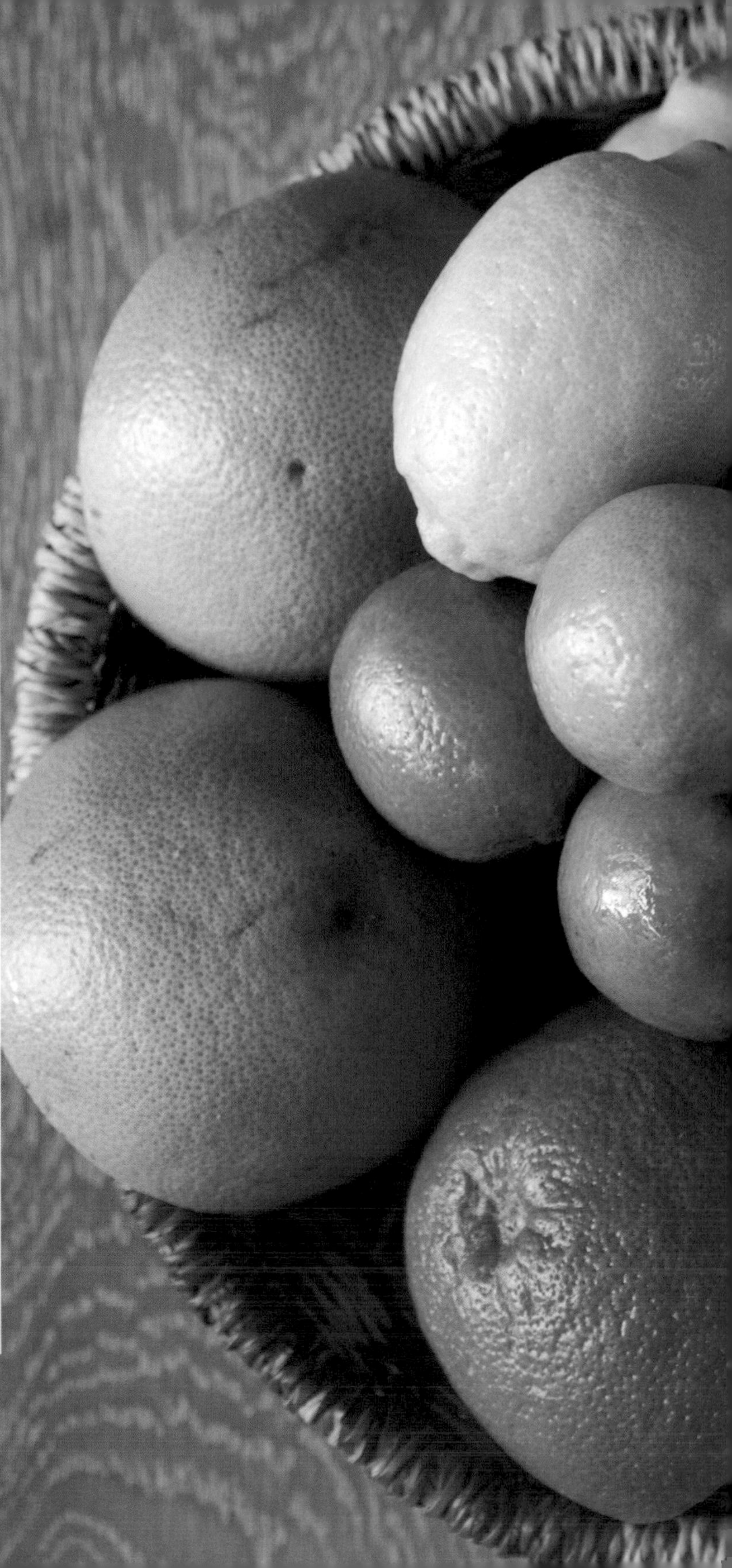

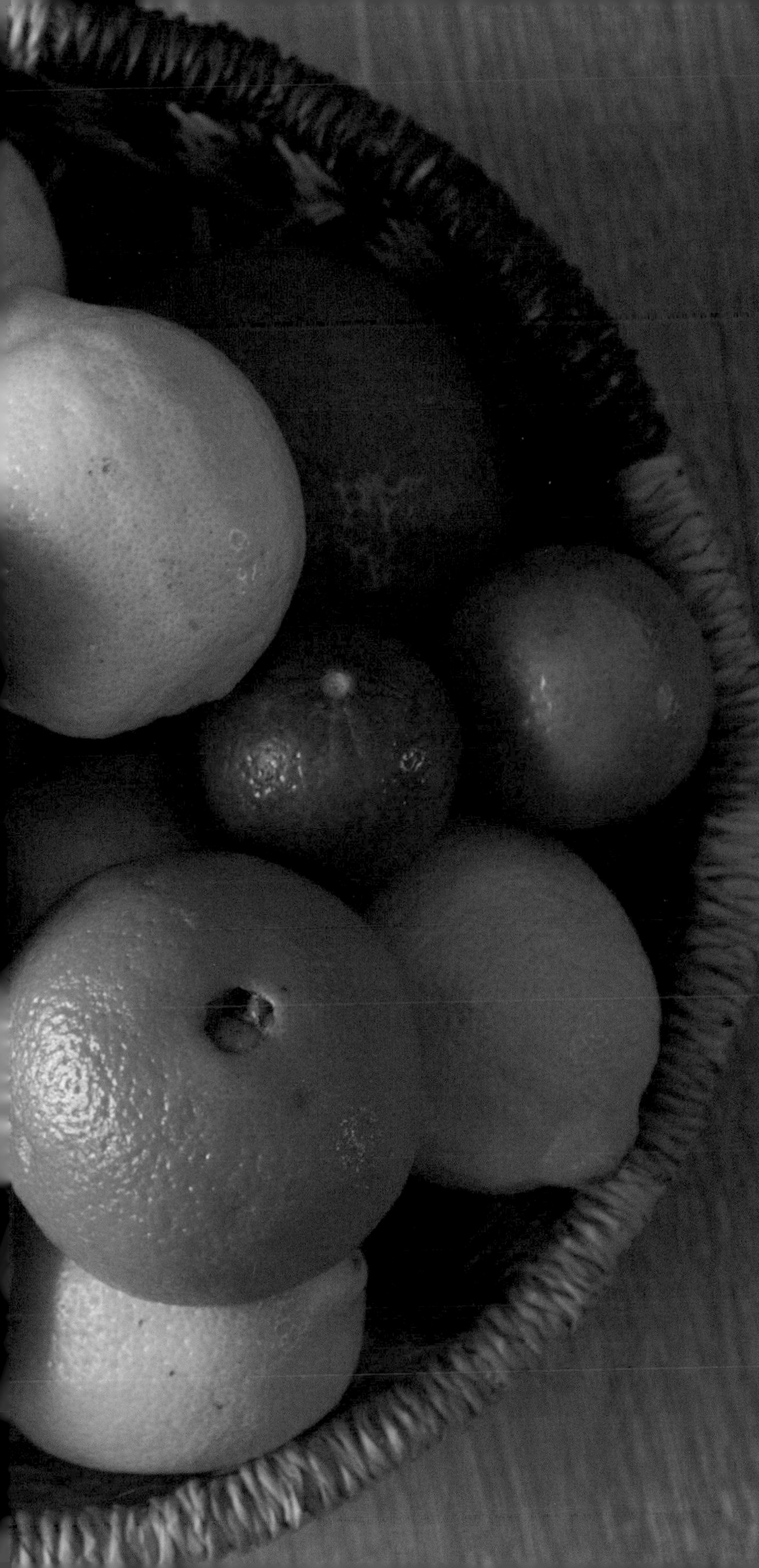

Make Me Smile

- 3 drops Bergamot essential oil
- 2 drops Douglas Fir essential oil
- 1 drop Juniper Berry essential oil
- 1 drop Myrrh essential oil

Island Sunset

- 4 drops Juniper Berry essential oil
- 2 drops Bergamot essential oil
- 2 drops Grapefruit essential oil
- 1 drop Ylang Ylang essential oil

Citrus Explosion

- 2 drops Wild Orange essential oil
- 1 drop Bergamot essential oil
- 1 drop Grapefruit essential oil
- 1 drop Lemon essential oil
- 1 drop Lime essential oil

19

Fall

These delightful scents will remind you of snuggly sweaters, warm scarves, and treats from Grandma baking in the oven.

Oatmeal Cookies

- 3 drops Wild Orange essential oil
- 2 drops Cassia essential oil
- 2 drops Cedarwood essential oil

Autumn in New York

- 3 drops Wild Orange essential oil
- 1 drop Clove essential oil
- 1 drop Geranium essential oil

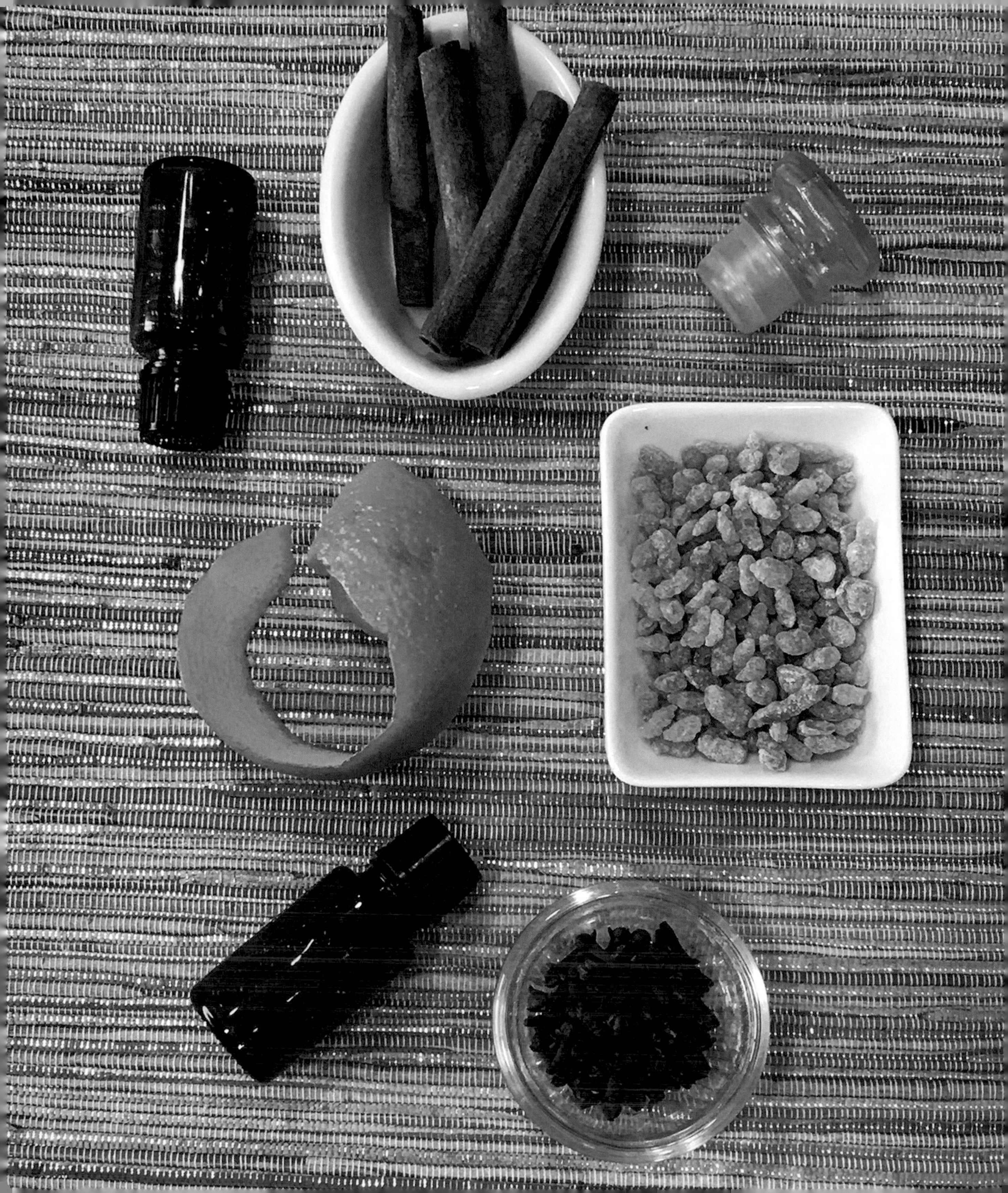

Citrus Spice

- 3 drops Wild Orange essential oil
- 1 drop Clove essential oil
- 1 drop Frankincense essential oil
- 1 drop Ginger essential oil

Autumn Rain

- 4 drops Grapefruit essential oil
- 2 drops Eucalyptus essential oil
- 1 drop Frankincense essential oil
- 1 drop Juniper Berry essential oil

Peace & Love

- 3 drops Patchouli essential oil
- 2 drops Bergamot essential oil
- 2 drops Cypress essential oil

Orange Pomander

- 3 drops Wild Orange essential oil
- 2 drops Clove essential oil
- 2 drops Rosemary essential oil

Crisp Autumn

- 3 drops Patchouli essential oil
- 3 drops Wild Orange essential oil
- 1 drop Clove essential oil

Pumpkin Pie

- 4 drops Cardamom essential oil
- 2 drops Cinnamon Bark essential oil
- 1 drop Wild Orange essential oil
- 1 drop Clove essential oil

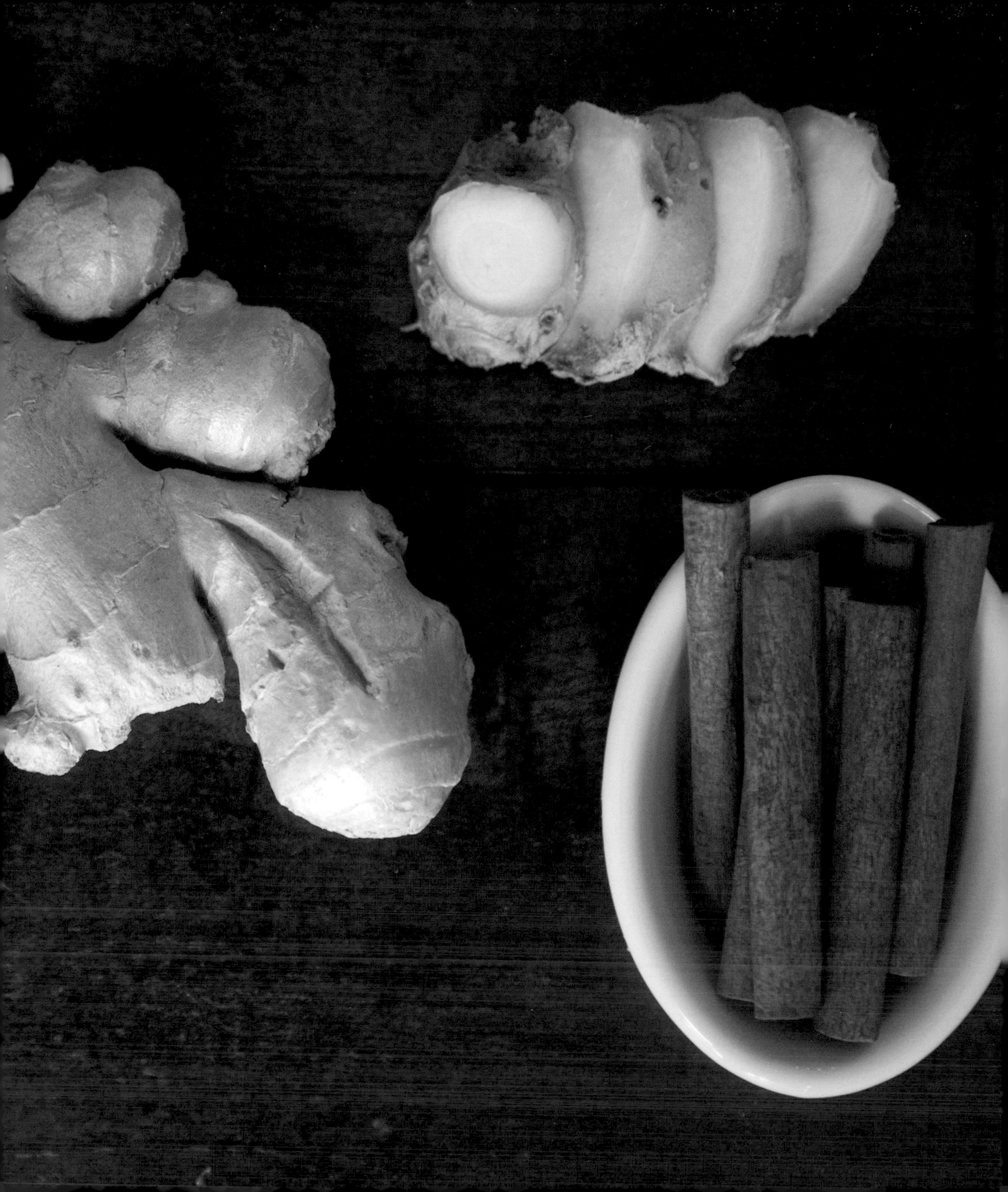

Be Thankful

- 2 drops Coriander essential oil
- 1 drop Cinnamon essential oil
- 1 drop Clove essential oil
- 1 drop Ginger essential oil

Spiced Chai

- 3 drops Cardamom essential oil
- 2 drops Cassia essential oil
- 2 drops Clove essential oil
- 1 drop Ginger essential oil

20

Winter

Baby, it's cold outside . . . but these diffuser blends will bring both warmth and spice to your home.

Peppermint Surprise

- 5 drops Peppermint essential oil
- 2 drops Ylang Ylang essential oil

Christmas Bells

- 2 drops Cinnamon essential oil
- 2 drops White Fir essential oil

Beat the Winter Blues

- 4 drops Lavender essential oil
- 4 drops Wild Orange essential oil
- 2 drops Frankincense essential oil

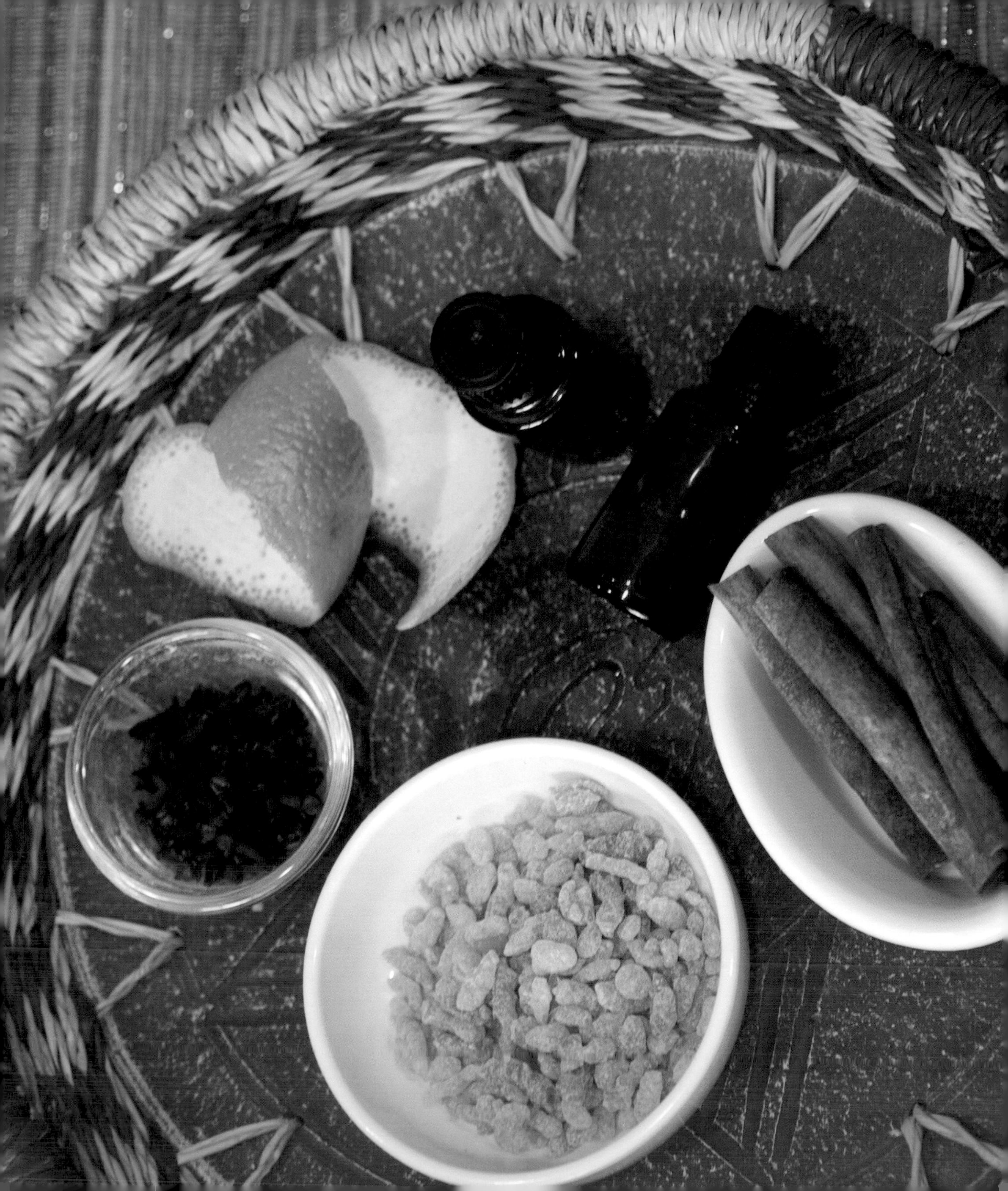

Holiday Spice

- 5 drops Bergamot essential oil
- 3 drops Cypress essential oil
- 3 drops Frankincense essential oil
- 3 drops Grapefruit essential oil
- 1 drop Ginger essential oil
- 1 drop Ylang Ylang essential oil

Winter Wonderland

- 3 drops White Fir essential oil
- 2 drops Cardamom essential oil
- 1 drop Clove essential oil

Three Gifts

- 3 drops Frankincense essential oil
- 2 drops Myrrh essential oil
- 1 drop Wild Orange essential oil

Happy Holidays

- 2 drops White Fir essential oil
- 2 drops Wild Orange essential oil
- 1 drop Wintergreen essential oil

Down in Yon Forest

- 3 drops Cedarwood essential oil
- 3 drops Pine essential oil
- 2 drops Blue Spruce essential oil

Rare & Precious

- 2 drops Cinnamon Bark essential oil
- 2 drops Frankincense essential oil
- 2 drops Myrrh essential oil
- 1 drop Rose essential oil

Into the Trees

- 3 drops Balsam Fir essential oil
- 3 drops Black Spruce essential oil
- 1 drop Cedarwood essential oil
- 1 drop Juniper Berry essential oil

Cinnamon Spice

- 4 drops Patchouli essential oil
- 2 drops Cinnamon Bark essential oil
- 3 drops Wild Orange essential oil
- 1 drop Clove essential oil
- 1 drop Ylang Ylang essential oil

21

Kids' Favorites

Kids love essential oils! Diffusers are safer than candles and chemical sprays, and these blends are bright, fresh scents that kids and adults will enjoy.

Root Beer

- 2 drops Wild Orange essential oil
- 2 drops Wintergreen essential oil
- 1 drop vanilla extract

Schoolhouse Rock

- 3 drops Douglas Fir essential oil
- 2 drops Lemon essential oil

Orange Crush

- 5 drops Wild Orange essential oil
- 2 drops Neroli essential oil
- 2 drops Petitgrain essential oil

Fruity Pebbles

- 2 drops Grapefruit essential oil
- 2 drops Lemon essential oil
- 1 drop Bergamot essential oil

Carnival Time

- 3 drops Lime essential oil
- 3 drops Wild Orange essential oil
- 2 drops Lemongrass essential oil

Snips and Snails

- 4 drops Spearmint essential oil
- 1 drop Fennel essential oil
- 1 drop Vetiver essential oil

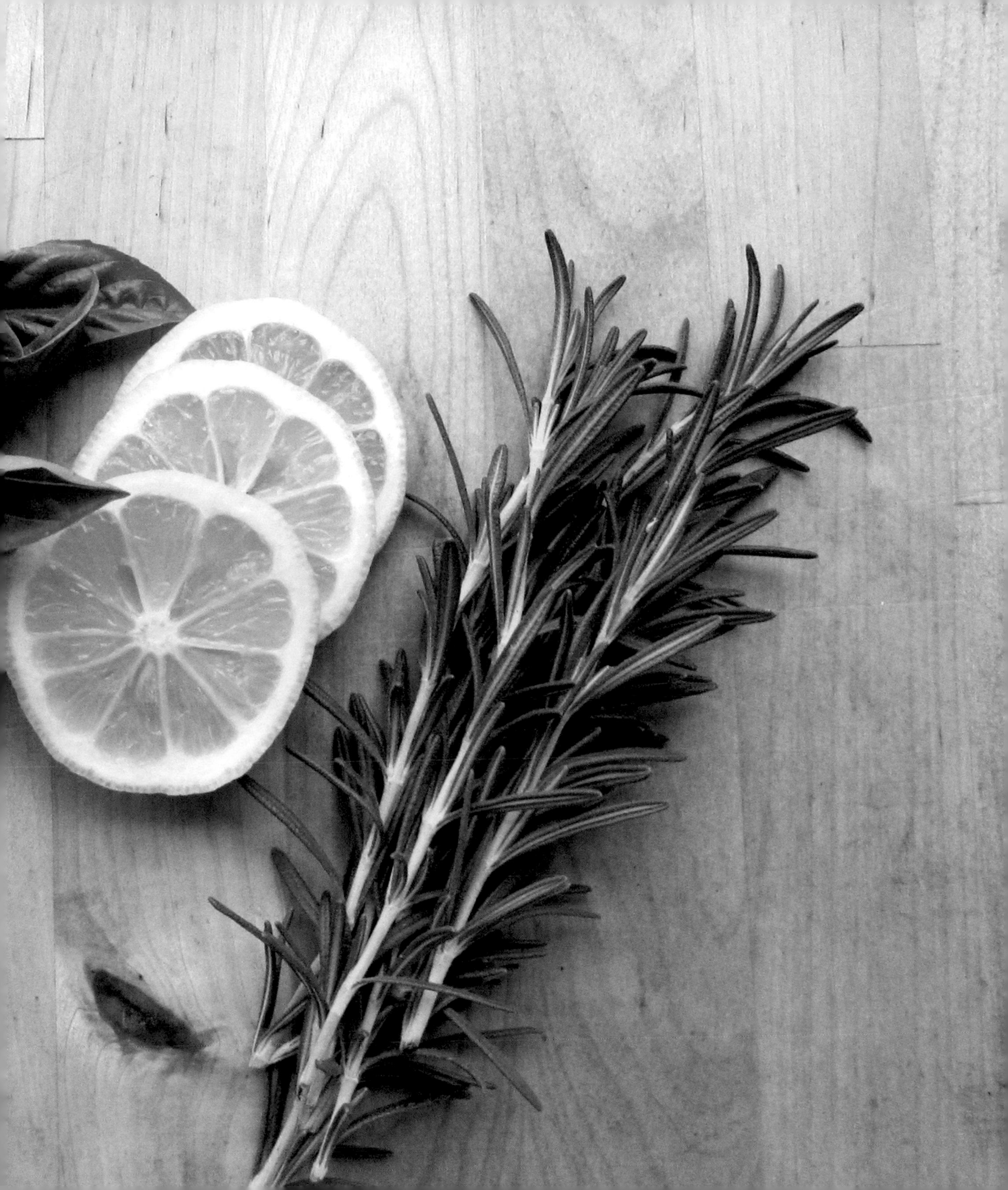

Homework Helper

- 4 drops Lemon essential oil
- 2 drops Basil essential oil
- 2 drops Rosemary essential oil

Four-Leaf Clover

- 2 drops Rosemary essential oil
- 2 drops Spearmint essential oil
- 1 drop Wild Orange essential oil

Citrus Twist

- 2 drops Bergamot essential oil
- 2 drops Petitgrain essential oil
- 2 drops Wild Orange essential oil

Bubble Gum

- 4 drops Grapefruit essential oil
- 2 drops Ylang Ylang essential oil
- 1 drop Eucalyptus essential oil

Fruit Loops

- 3 drops Bergamot essential oil
- 3 drops Grapefruit essential oil
- 3 drops Lemongrass essential oil

Jelly Beans

- 3 drops Wild Orange essential oil
- 2 drops Juniper Berry essential oil
- 1 drop Lemongrass essential oil
- 1 drop Vanilla extract

Key Lime Pie

- 4 drops Lime essential oil
- 1 drop Lavender essential oil
- 1 drop Lemon essential oil
- 1 drop Vanilla extract

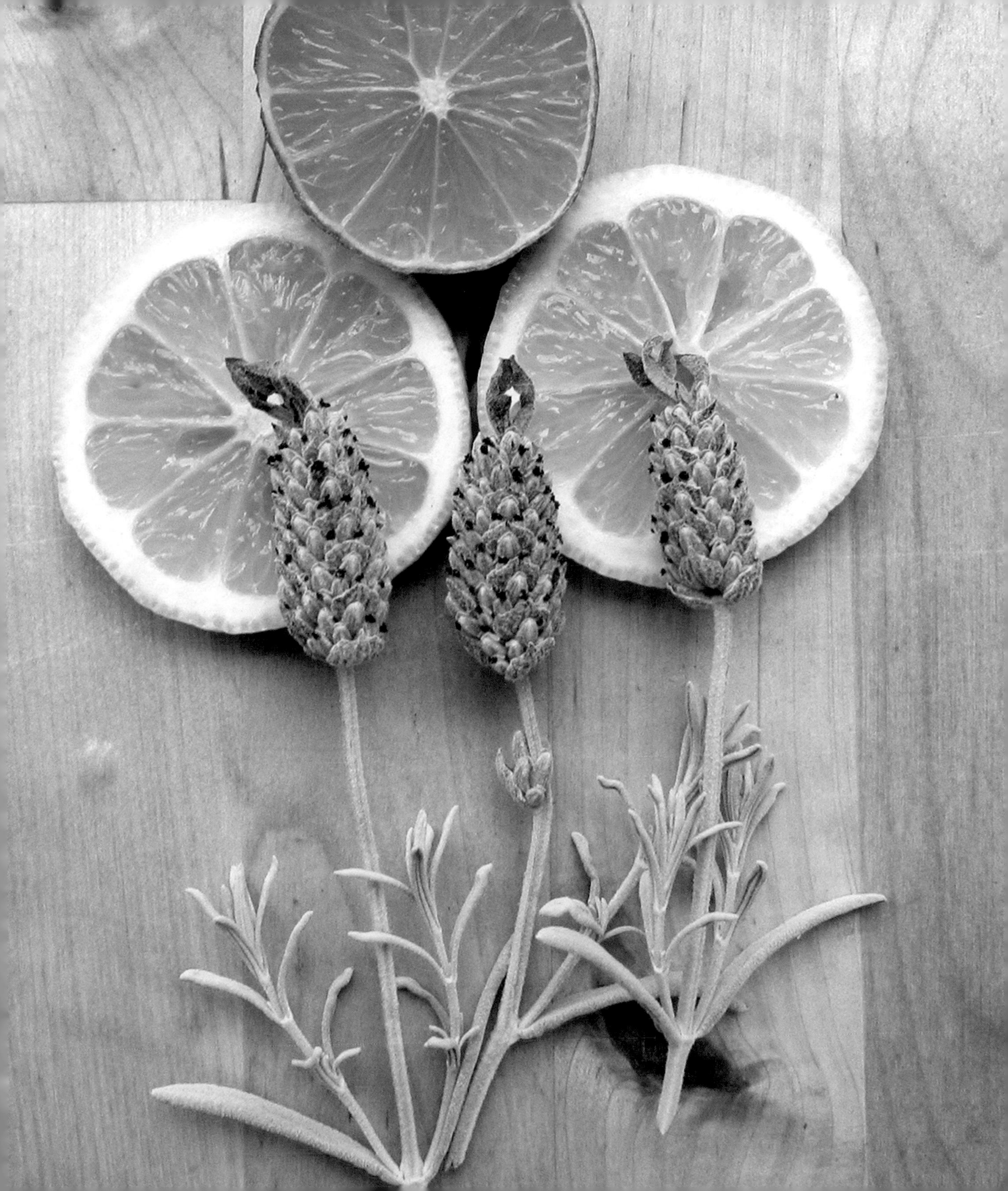

About the Author

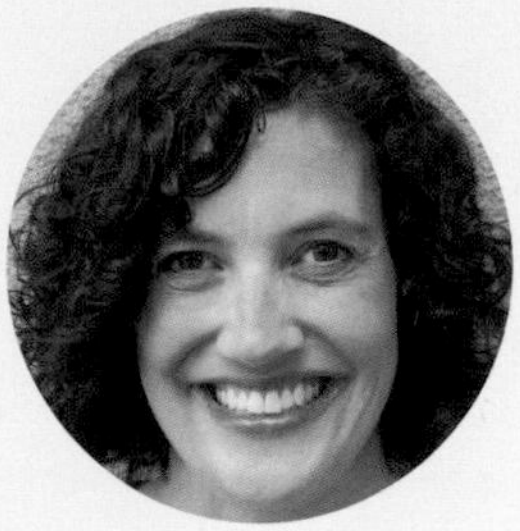

Pam Farley lives her motto of "make it, don't buy it" every day as the founder of BrownThumbMama.com, a website dedicated to healthy living, natural eating, and attempted gardening.

A former corporate writer, she ditched the cubicle in 2015. Now she spends her time working from home with her family, growing vegetables in her front yard, teaching about essential oils, and avoiding housework.

You can learn more about the premium essential oils she uses and recommends at www.BrownThumbMama.com/oils.

brown thumb mama

Natural living. Healthy eating. Attempted gardening.

Index